ENNIS AND NANCY HAM LIBRARY
ROCHESTER COLLEGE
800 WEST AVON ROAD
ROCHESTER HILLS, MI 48307

THE MILK OF PARADISE

THE MILK OF PARADISE

The Effect of Opium Visions on the Works of DeQuincey, Crabbe, Francis Thompson, and Coleridge

BY

M. H. ABRAMS

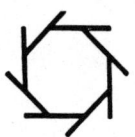

1971

OCTAGON BOOKS
New York

Copyright 1934 by the President and Fellows of Harvard College
Copyright © 1962 by M. H. Abrams
Author's note copyright © 1970 by M. H. Abrams

Reprinted 1971

by special arrangement with Harvard University Press, and M. H. Abrams, and Harper & Row, Publishers, Incorporated

OCTAGON BOOKS
A Division of Farrar, Straus & Giroux, Inc.
19 Union Square West
New York, N. Y. 10003

Library of Congress Catalog Card Number: 79-120223

ISBN-0-374-90028-0

Printed in U.S.A. by
NOBLE OFFSET PRINTERS, INC.
NEW YORK 3, N. Y.

TO MY TUTOR
ARTHUR COLBY SPRAGUE

"For he on honey-dew hath fed,
And drunk the milk of Paradise."

KUBLA KHAN

CONTENTS

Author's Note, 1969	ix
Preface	xv
THE MILK OF PARADISE	1
Appendix: Coleridge's Use of Opium before 1798	51
Notes	61
Bibliography	81
Appendix to the Perennial Library edition:	87
—George Crabbe,	
"The World of Dreams"	89
"Sir Eustace Grey"	99
—Francis Thompson,	
"Finis Coronat Opus"	113

AUTHOR'S NOTE

This little book began as an essay in a sophomore survey course in English literature at Harvard, and two years later was expanded to its present form as a senior thesis for honors. In the early 1930's the subject of the effect of opium on imagination was an exotic one, which appealed to an undergraduate author precisely because it lay outside the realm of his conceivable experience. The passage of some thirty-five years has made the subject unexpectedly topical, now that drugs have become a standard means to force an "expansion of consciousness" by a direct assault upon the nervous system.

Were I writing this essay now, I would sharpen the discrimination between various modes of experience affected by opium, which in the present text are sometimes grouped under the general term "vision" or "dream." The drug may intensify or distort sense-perception, especially audition and the visual apprehension of space, structure, light, and color. To be distinguished from

AUTHOR'S NOTE

such perception of outer phenomena is the reverie or intense daydream—the sequence of fantasied images and experiences in the partly autonomous and partly controlled states of the waking mind which De Quincey, in discussing his opium experiences, called "trances, or profoundest reveries." In a note on a manuscript of "Kubla Khan" which was not printed until 1934, just after this essay had been published, Coleridge wrote that the poem was "composed in a sort of Reverie brought on by two grains of Opium." In attributing the genesis of his poem to a play of the waking fantasy Coleridge was more precise than in his later statement (in the Preface of 1816) that "Kubla Khan" was composed "in a profound sleep, at least of the external senses," during which "all the images rose up before him as *things*, with a parallel production of the correspondent expressions, without any sensation or consciousness of effort." Both sense-perception and reverie are in turn to be distinguished from dreams, nightmares, and hallucinations. These last phenomena—the subject-matter of De Quincey's "The Pains of Opium" and Coleridge's "The Pains

AUTHOR'S NOTE

of Sleep"—are associated with deep addiction to opium, and are experienced especially during periods of deprivation or total abstinence.

I would also, if I were writing now, be more tentative in tracing opium experience in products of the literary imagination, for such matters do not permit certainty, but only various degrees of probability. Above all I would put greater stress on the brevity of the period of euphoria in opium addiction. In a very short time De Quincey's "The Pleasures of Opium" become merely negative, the assuagement of a savage craving, and the drug is recognized, in Coleridge's bitter words, as this "dirty business of Laudanum . . . this *free-agency-annihilating* Poison."

In *Coleridge, Opium and 'Kubla Khan'* (Chicago, 1953) Elisabeth Schneider put in question Coleridge's account of the origin of "Kubla Khan" in an opium reverie, marshalling evidence from recent medical reports on opium addiction to support her claim that the drug does not greatly affect sense-perception and that it neither stimulates nor alters the ordinary process of

AUTHOR'S NOTE

reveries and dreams. This type of evidence, however, is of dubious probative value with respect to the writers and writings treated in this essay. Modern investigators deal mainly with confirmed addicts who inject into the bloodstream morphine or heroin, which are alkaloid derivatives of opium; the authors I deal with all drank laudanum, which is raw or partially refined opium dissolved in alcohol, and some of the experiences they represent occurred in an early stage of their resort to the drug. The social and psychological ambiance—which undoubtedly affects the nature of the experience with drugs—has also undergone a drastic change. Indulgence in opium is now a furtive, and in the United States a criminal activity, and often constitutes a deliberate gesture of defiance against society. Through much of the nineteenth century, however, opium was not only readily and legally available, but was recommended by reigning medical opinion for an enormous variety of ailments from earliest infancy on; opium-taking was subject to no sanction outside the judgment and conscience of

AUTHOR'S NOTE

the taker; and those who indulged often had extravagant expectations about the psychic effects of the drug. Most importantly, as De Quincey early pointed out, "If a man 'whose talk is of oxen' should become an opium-eater, the probability is, that (if he is not too dull to dream at all)— he will dream about oxen." "Habitually to dream magnificently, a man must have a constitutional determination to reverie." Anyone who investigates the effects of opium must take into account the differences—in sensory endowment, the tendency to fantasy, the proclivity to subtle self-analysis, the wealth of available literary memories, and the power of the trained imagination—between the representative addict who turns up in a modern clinic and Crabbe, Coleridge, De Quincey, and Francis Thompson. In a more recent book, *Opium and the Romantic Imagination* (Berkeley: University of California Press, 1968), Alethea Hayter examined thoroughly both the medical and psychological evidence about opium and the writings of addicted authors. Her conclusion was that indulgence in laudanum tends

AUTHOR'S NOTE

to effect characteristic patterns of imagery which are recognizable in a number of works of the literary imagination.

The books by Miss Schneider[1] and Miss Hayter are the only comprehensive studies of the effects of opium on literature which have appeared since 1934.[2] Their texts, together with the notes and bibliographies, provide a convenient survey, to date, of the medical, biographical, and critical studies of individual authors who have drunk the milk of a dubious paradise.

M. H. ABRAMS

Cornell University
June, 1969

---

[1] Elisabeth Schneider, *Coleridge, Opium and 'Kubla Khan,'* Chicago: University of Chicago Press, 1953.

[2] A recent study of the effect of drugs on French literature is Emanuel J. Mickel, Jr., *The Artificial Paradises in French Literature,* Chapel Hill: The University of North Carolina Press, 1969.

PREFACE

Four eminent English authors were addicted to opium. Each author spent a considerable part of his life in a dream world which differs amazingly from that in which we live. Each author utilized the imagery from these dreams in his literary creations, and sometimes, under the direct inspiration of opium, achieved his best writing. Thus, a knowledge of the opium world these authors inhabited is essential to a complete understanding of their work.

In the cases where critics have not entirely neglected this factor, their analysis of opium effects is too often a flight of conjecture unimpeded by any burden of definite knowledge. Strangely enough, although "there is hardly a more difficult chapter in the whole of pharmacology than . . . a thoroughly exact analysis of the effects of drugs,"* this is just the field wherein each man seems to consider himself expert. When a critic of established reputation is misled into characterizing all of Coleridge's finest poems as "the

* Louis Lewin, *Phantastica*, London, 1931, Preface, p. x.

PREFACE

chance brain-blooms of a season of physiological ecstasy,"* it is time to examine the facts. Accordingly, I have based my investigation of the nature of opium phenomena on the statements of habituates and the findings of psychological authorities. Moreover, since to postulate addiction to opium merely from the "abnormality" of a man's work, although the usual method, is illogical, my approach to each of the authors under consideration is biographical.

Limitations of the length allowed for this thesis have imposed limitations in subject. I have dealt with no drug but opium, except in a passing reference in the Notes. Foreign authors I have had to omit; and of English authors I have been able to treat at length only those four whose long addiction to the drug is certain: DeQuincey, Crabbe, Francis Thompson, and Coleridge. Even with these men, it has been necessary to cut down evidence to a minimum, but indications for further investigation will be found in the Notes. There is no definite proof of addiction to opium in the lives of James Thomson and

* John Mackinnon Robertson, *New Essays towards a Critical Method*, London, 1897, p. 190.

PREFACE

Poe.* In their works, too, indications of the influence of alcohol are so strong that it would be difficult to distinguish any possible effect of opium.

Since the date of the inception of Coleridge's opium habit is necessary for a determination of the influence of the drug on his great creative period, I have gathered in an appendix all the evidence available on this agitated question.

To Professor Lowes I owe a great debt for the material on Coleridge in *The Road to Xanadu*, and for access to his photostatic reproductions of Coleridge's manuscript Note Book. To Dr. David Worcester I am grateful for the benefit of his authoritative investigations on James Thomson. I wish to express my appreciation also to Professor Edmund B. Delabarre, of the Psychology Department of Brown University, and to Dr. Beebe-Center, for guidance in matters connected with the subject of narcotic phenomena.

* The more important books which I have consulted are listed in the bibliography.

THE MILK OF PARADISE

THE MILK OF PARADISE

W<small>HEN</small> H<small>OMER</small> sang of "the drug to heal all pain and anger, and bring forgetfulness of every sorrow," [1] he heralded a long succession of poets who paid tribute to the enchantment of opium. Vergil knew the "poppies soaked with the sleep of Lethe"; [2] and in his *Aeneid*, the dragon which protects the distant Hesperides succumbs to this chastening gift of Somnus, god of sleep.[3] The great English poets, too, felt the poppy's spell. Chaucer twice mentions opium; [4] Shakespeare knows the effect of "the drowsy syrups of the world"; [5] Milton recalls Homer with

> The Nepenthes which the wife of Thone
> In Egypt gave to Jove-born Helena.[6]

These poets were allured by the mystery inherent in the golden drug of Asia; but when English authors, early in the nineteenth century, actually took opium themselves, they were inspired to ecstasies. "A spot of enchantment, a green spot of fountain and flowers and trees in the very heart of a waste of sands!" [7] So Coleridge hailed it, and found therein a refuge from the turmoil of aspiration and disillusion at the turn of the century. DeQuincey apostrophized the drug more grandly: "Just, subtle, and all-conquering opium!" . . . "*Eloquent* opium!" For he saw not only a sanctuary, but a new sphere opened to his imagination in the glowing splendors it built "upon the bosom of darkness, out of the fantastic imagery of the brain." [8]

The great gift of opium to these men was access to a new world as different from this as Mars may be; and one which ordinary mortals, hindered by terrestrial conceptions, can never, from mere description, quite comprehend. It is a world of twisted, exquisite experience, sensuous and intellectual; of "music like a perfume," and "sweet light golden with audible odors exquisite," [9] where color is a symphony, and one can hear the walk of an insect on the ground, the bruising of a flower.[10] Above all, in this enchanted land man is freed at last from those petty bonds upon which Kant insists: space and time. Space is amplified to such proportions that, to writer after writer, "infinity" is the only word adequate to compass it. More striking still, man escapes at last from the life of a transiency lamented by poets since time immemorial, and approaches immortality as closely as he ever can in this world; for he experiences, almost literally, eternity. This is not the abstract "eternity" of the mystic, not Vaughan's vision of "a great ring of pure and endless light," but the duration of an actual, continuous experience so long that DeQuincey throws up his hands in an attempt to measure it by mundane standards:

In valuing the *virtual* time lived during some dreams, the measurement by generations is ridiculous—by millenia is ridiculous; by aeons, I should say, if aeons were more determinate, would also be ridiculous.[11]

This fantastic land is not the fleeting shadow of an ordinary dream, but is a reality nearly as vivid as actual experience.[12] The important and almost neglected fact is that in "the well of memory" the fragments of this land assume as legitimate a place as any recollections from life. When the poet's selective spirit hovers over the well, these images rise to the surface as readily as any others, to be incorporated in his creation side by side with the scenes from everyday life.

THE MILK OF PARADISE

To reconstruct the world of dreams vividly enough to distinguish its fragments in the works of men who have roamed its exotic paths is the hazardous task I have undertaken.

In all the writings of the four men with whom I am concerned, DeQuincey's *Confessions of an English Opium-Eater* is the only acknowledged description of opium visions. Coleridge so denoted only the passing reference, in his letters, to the "green spot of fountain and trees"; we know of Thompson's recourse to opium only through the indirect testimony of Everard Meynell; [13] and if it were not for an incidental acknowledgment by Crabbe's son,[14] and a friend's hasty jotting on a copy of his poems,[15] Crabbe's addiction might have escaped notice altogether.

Whether or not the impulse which caused DeQuincey to break this bond of silence was his avowed intention to be "useful and instructive," [16] his *Confessions* may serve as a key to the mysteries of the opium world. That his descriptions of the effects of opium are authentic is verified, not only by his own reiterated insistence,[17] but by the fact that psychological investigators still draw on the *Confessions* for data.

DeQuincey, an Oxford student of nineteen, took opium for the first time in 1804, under coercion of excruciating rheumatic pains of head and face.[18] In accordance with accepted medical opinion, an acquaintance recommended opium, and DeQuincey tried it without question.[19] So enticing was the "abyss of divine enjoyment" revealed to him that for ten years he tasted the delights of the drug with indulgences at three-week intervals,[20] until in 1813 an "appalling irritation of the stomach" led to a daily resort to opium, and the addiction which lasted until his death. As with other authors, dreams of horror after long consumption of opium, rather than the pleasures experienced at the inception of the habit, stimulated most his desire for literary expression.[21] The visions described in the *Confessions* are the "Iliad of woes" attendant upon a futile struggle against the drug;[22] the "pleasures of opium" are lauded, but with no specific detail.[23]

The first symptom upon which DeQuincey comments, he calls "the re-awakening of a state of eye oftentimes incident to childhood": an endless succession of scenes passing through his mind; the subject, perhaps, voluntarily chosen, but its evolution out of control.[24] Havelock Ellis, in *The World of Dreams*, also remarks upon this "constant succession of self-evolving visual imagery," and felicitously likens it "to the images produced by the kaleidoscope."[25] Dupouy, describing the same effect in greater detail, notes, too, that "les pensées et les tableaux se succèdent sans arrêt, faisant défiler les vies, les générations, et les siècles."[26]

DeQuincey then analyzes the distorted perceptions which seem to characterize all opium visions, whether of pleasure or of pain, the enormous extension of space and time.

> Space swelled, and was amplified to an extent of unutterable and self-repeating infinity. This disturbed me very much less than the vast expansion of time. Sometimes I seemed to have lived for seventy or a hundred years in one night; nay, sometimes had feelings representative of a duration far beyond the limits of any human experience.[27]

"Le temps n'existe plus, l'espace est illimité," Dupouy corroborates;[28] and adds that if the addict imagines himself on a lake, "ce lac est immense, sans fond ni bournes; les montagnes qui l'entourent sont d'une hauteur prodigieuse, et lui-même met un temps illimité, 10,000, 20,000 ans à en accomplir la traversée." [29]

In the early stages, these exalted splendors of DeQuincey's dreams were chiefly architectural, "such pomp of cities and palaces as never yet was beheld by the waking eye, unless in the clouds." To these succeeded "dreams of lakes and silvery expanses of water," which, by the alchemy of opium, were soon amplified: "From translucent lakes, shining like mirrors, they became seas and oceans." [30]

Now began the affliction so horrible that it has impressed itself more deeply than any other dream experience on the work of every opium author. DeQuincey calls it "the tyranny of the human face"; but this manifestation is only one aspect of a many-sided evil, the delusion of pursuit and persecution:

Upon the rocking waters of the ocean the human face began to reveal itself; the sea appeared paved with innumerable faces, upturned to the heavens; faces, imploring, wrathful, despairing; faces that surged upwards by thousands, by myriads, by generations.[31]

THE MILK OF PARADISE

But the many faces soon gave place to one, that of a Malay who, like a genie conjured by Aladdin's lamp, had appeared one day at DeQuincey's peaceful country cottage.[32] Fearfully metamorphosed from that harmless vagrant, the dream fiend transports his helpless victim, night after endless night, through fantastic scenes which are the accumulations of all DeQuincey's Asiatic memories, fused under the unifying principle of guilt and horror:

> I was stared at, hooted at, grinned at, chattered at, by monkeys, by paraquets, by cockatoos. I ran into pagodas, and was fixed for centuries at the summit, or in secret rooms. . . . I fled from the wrath of Brama through all the forests of Asia; Vishnu hated me; Seeva lay in wait for me. . . . I had done a deed, they said, which the ibis and the crocodile trembled at. Thousands of years I lived and was buried in stone coffins, with mummies and sphinxes, in narrow chambers at the heart of eternal pyramids. I was kissed with cancerous kisses, by crocodiles, and was laid, confounded with all unutterable abortions, amongst reeds and Nilotic mud.[33]

Note here the kaleidoscopic rush of scenes, and that omnipresent sensation of distorted time — "fixed for *centuries*," "*thousands* of years," "*eternal* pyramids." And later in the same vision, "Over every form, and threat, and punishment, and dim sightless incarceration, brooded a killing sense of *eternity* and *infinity*." [34]

Into these dreams, although all before had been "moral and spiritual terrors," now entered circumstances of "physical horror":

> Here the main agents were ugly birds, or snakes, or crocodiles. . . . All the feet of the tables, sofas, &c., soon became instinct with life: the abominable head of the crocodile, and his leering eyes, looked out at me, multiplied into ten thousand repetitions; and I stood loathing and fascinated. [35]

In the original manuscript of the *Confessions* appeared another passage which, although immediately cancelled by the writer, has since been published in Garnett's reprint.[36] The dreams become so terrifying, that, DeQuincey says:

> At length I grew afraid to sleep, and I shrank from it as from the most savage torture. Often I fought with my drowsiness, and kept it aloof by sitting up the whole night and the following day.[37]

Yet he had to sleep at times; and turning back to the published *Confessions*, we find a new series of visions, beginning with the

lovely one of the "Sunday morning in May."
DeQuincey is standing at what seems the
door of his actual cottage; but, with the
usual exaltation of space, "the mountains
were raised to more than Alpine height, and
there was interspace far larger between them
of savannahs and forest lawns." Then suddenly "the scene is an Oriental one . . . and
at a vast distance are visible, as a stain upon
the horizon, the domes and cupolas of a great
city." [38]

There follows the breathless description of
the finding, under Judean palms, of Ann, the
forlorn little prostitute who had befriended
him in London seventeen years before. Another turn of the kaleidoscope, vapors roll in,
and DeQuincey is back in London. And
again a flux of scene, heralded by the welling
of sounds on a drugged mentality, as he
hears

> music of preparation and of awakening suspense. The undulations of fast-gathering tumults
> . . . gave the feeling of a multitudinous movement, of infinite cavalcades filing off, and the
> tread of innumerable armies.[39]

As the view unrolls, the scene again contorts into one of horror, with "darkness and lights; tempests and human faces." Ann reappears, but only for a moment, then — "everlasting farewells!" And as the sound is reverberated — again and again, "everlasting farewells!" — he 'awakes in struggles, and cries aloud, "I will sleep no more!"' [40]

To those who know George Crabbe as a sedate and dignified ecclesiastic, his classification with the comparatively disreputable DeQuincey, Thompson, and Coleridge may seem a bit incongruous, even irreverent; but a touch of the poppy makes the world of poets kin. In the biography written by Crabbe's son occurs a paragraph to the significance of which most critics have been as blind as was the author.[41] After Crabbe had experienced a fainting spell in 1790,[42] a certain Dr. Club was called who "saw through the case with great judgment," and declared, to quote the son:

"Let the digestive organs bear the whole blame; you must take opiates." [43] From that time his health began to amend rapidly, . . . a rare effect of opium; . . . and to a constant but slightly increasing dose of it may be attributed his long and generally healthy life.[44]

From Crabbe himself we learn that this "constant but slightly increasing dose" finally resulted in the usual dreams of horror. What is apparently only one of many similar experiences is narrated in his journal of 1817:

> For the first time these many nights, I was incommoded by dreams, such as would cure vanity for a time in any mind where they could gain admission.... Asleep, all was misery and degradation, not my own only, but of those who had been. — That horrible image of servility and baseness — that mercenary and commercial manner! [45]

The poet Fitzgerald, who in a twenty-two year friendship with Crabbe's son had learned much about the father's habits,[46] adds to the list of evidence. In Fitzgerald's copy of Crabbe's poems, Ainger informs us,

> there is a MS note, not signed "G. C.," and therefore Fitzgerald's own. It runs thus: "It (the opium) probably influenced his dreams, for better or worse." To this Fitzgerald significantly adds, "see also the *World of Dreams,* and his *Eustace Grey.*" [47]

The opening stanza of the "World of Dreams"[48] confirms Fitzgerald's hypothesis that the visions described in the poem are of opium origin. The division of dreams into extremes of pleasure and pain at once echoes the keynote of DeQuincey's *Confessions*:

> And is thy soul so wrapt in sleep?
> Thy senses, thy affections, fled?
> No play of fancy thine, to keep
> Oblivion from that grave, thy bed?
> Then art thou but the breathing dead:
> I envy, but I pity too:
> The bravest may *my* terrors dread,
> The happiest fain *my* joys pursue. . . .
>
> I feel such bliss, I fear such pain;
> But all is gloom, or all is gay,
> Soon as th' ideal World I gain.

This "ideal World" of Crabbe's diluted phraseology, it soon becomes evident, is the same twisted world of opium into which DeQuincey had entered. With characteristic phantasmagoric succession, the restless scene shifts from "the wicked city's vilest street" to "a noble mansion," to "far-off rivers"; then, after a flash of the sea, to the land again; on and on, fading, receding, expanding, brightening.

In spite of DeQuincey's failure to give a detailed picture of his visions of pleasure, the following scene is enough like Cole-

THE MILK OF PARADISE

ridge's "green spot of fountain and flowers and trees" to indicate its type. The force of this description is lost upon those unacquainted with the usual cold restraint of Crabbe's style:

> A garden this? Oh! lovely breeze!
> Oh! flowers that with such freshness bloom!
> Flowers shall I call such forms as these;
> Or this delicious air perfume?
> Oh! this from better worlds must come;
> On earth such beauty who can meet?

Then occurs the illusion of flight, which, though new to this investigation, is an authenticated characteristic of narcotic experience: [49]

> 'Tis easier now to soar than run;
> Up! Up! — we neither tire nor fall.
> Children of dust, be yours to crawl
> On the vile earth!

Unfortunately, these delights are soon metamorphosed into the familiar hallucinations of persecution and horror, crowded with "black Enemies," in which "the darkbrow'd throng" jostle a "female fiend" with "tainted bosom bare" and "eye of stone." Time is extended in "that sad, last, long endless day!" And again we hear the welling of noise, like DeQuincey's "undulations of fast-gathering tumults":

> Heavens! how mighty is the throng,
> Voices humming like a hive!

Although the Orient held the greatest terror for DeQuincey, Crabbe, like a true eighteenth-century man of letters, seems to have feared most the horrors of the Gothic. He is brought into a "Gothic hall," and seated with

> Kings, Caliphs, Kaisers, — silent all;
> Pale as the dead; enrobed and tall,
> Majestic, frozen, solemn, still;
> They wake my fears, my wits appal,
> And with both scorn and terror fill.

Strikingly close to similar experiences upon which DeQuincey had commented [50] is the reappearance in Crabbe's dreams of the friends of his childhood, "all whom he loved and thought them dead." And as DeQuincey had met Ann in his dreams, so Crabbe sees

> One, the fairest, best,
> Among them — ever-welcome guest! . . .
>
> Speak to me! speak! that I may know
> I am thus happy! — dearest, speak!

But, as in DeQuincey's dream, the dear forms disappear in the tumult, the terrors become ever more unbearable, until Crabbe, by a last desperate struggle, frees himself; and so perfect is the illusion, we can almost hear him crying, as DeQuincey had done, "I will sleep no more!"

"Sir Eustace Grey," composed by Crabbe fifteen years after he had begun to take opium,[51] again confirms Fitzgerald's judgment. This time the opium phenomena are not merely described, but are placed in a framework of plot designed to account for their peculiarities: a madman's recital of the fiendish persecution attending him since the murder of his young wife's paramour. We may detect the line, I feel certain, where the transcriptions from Crabbe's dreams begin:

> Soon came a voice! I felt it come;
> "Full be his cup, with evil fraught,
> "Demons his guides, and death his doom!" [52]

Immediately follows the usual eternal and kaleidoscopically varied persecution. Even the Malay who had been the supervisor of DeQuincey's tortures finds his counterpart in Crabbe's "two fiends":

THE MILK OF PARADISE

> Then was I cast from out my state,
> Two fiends of darkness led my way;
> They waked me early, watch'd me late,
> My dread by night, my plague by day!

Space is again amplified in the "boundless plain," "vast ruins," and "pillars and pediments sublime"; and, as usual, the bonds of time are burst:

> There was I fix'd, I know not how,
> Condemn'd for untold years to stay:
> Yet years were not; — one dreadful *Now*
> Endured no change of night or day.

As DeQuincey had been fixed for centuries at the summit of pagodas, so:

> They hung me on a bough so small,
> The rook could build her nest no higher;
> They fix'd me on the trembling ball
> That crowns the steeple's quiv'ring spire.

Interminably, the tormenting fiends continue their savage game. Sir Eustace is pursued through a "bleak and frozen land," riveted to a tombstone, placed upon a shaking fen" where "danced the moon's deceitful light," hung upon "the ridgy steep of cliffs," plunged "below the billowy deep"; then abruptly, again like a sudden *awakening* from a nightmare, comes the call of grace to release him from his tortures. But before I leave the poem, one bit of imagery I wish to emphasize because of its appearance in later writers:

> They placed me where those streamers play,
> Those nimble beams of brilliant light;
> It would the stoutest heart dismay,
> To see, to feel that dreadful sight:
> So swift, so pure, so cold, so bright,
> They pierced my frame with icy wound;
> And all that half-year's polar night,
> Those dancing streamers wrapp'd me round.

That DeQuincey made no special comment on abnormal light perception in a drugged state does not prove he noticed none. It may rather be the result of an innate lack of sensitivity to light. Although ordinary dreams are prevailingly gray in color,[53] in opium visions, as Beaudelaire affirms, occur "des échappées magnifiques, gorgées de lumière et de couleur."[54] Dupouy, moreover, describes a sensitivity of the eye so great that it translates vivid ocular impressions in terms of actual physical pain.[55] Thus Crabbe could speak of *feeling* light as an "icy wound."

It seems strange that Saintsbury could describe as an exponent of "the style of drab stucco" the author of the stanza above,[56] yet this statement is not unfair when applied to almost any of Crabbe's work except the two poems most critics neglect: "The World of Dreams" and "Sir Eustace Grey." Significantly, these same two poems and no others that I could discover describe the world of Crabbe's opium dreams.[57] These poems offer, therefore, an unexampled opportunity to observe the effect of opium on that mysterious phenomenon, poetic inspiration. On two occasions something happened to Crabbe which "set the winds of inspiration blowing," [58] tore him loose from the clutch of the heroic couplet, and caused the employment, in these two poems only, of an eight-line stanza with interlacing rhymes, almost as intricate as the Spenserian.[59] This same force, in at least a score of stanzas of "Sir Eustace Grey," freed Crabbe's language from the restraint of eighteenth-century poetic diction, and gave it a simplicity and inevitability which suggest Coleridge's "Ancient Mariner." With the evidence presented, is there much doubt that this stimulus, which incited Crabbe to dash off "Sir Eustace Grey" in a single night,[60] is the vivid recollection of an opium dream?

However admonitory were DeQuincey's intentions, the list of addicts introduced to opium by his *Confessions* is a long one, and extends even to the present day.[61] The last gift that Francis Thompson received from his mother was a copy of the *Confessions*. He was then, in 1879, a misfit medical student wandering ill and friendless in dingy Manchester.[62] In this condition, and under the stimulation of DeQuincey's rhapsodies, a resort to opium was almost inevitable.[63] "Giver of life, death, peace, distress" Thompson later termed his mother,[64] and thereby summed up the conflicting doles of the drug to which she had unsuspectingly introduced him.

Thompson rarely alluded to this surrender, but we find the records of his opium addiction in the biography written by his friend, Everard Meynell. In 1882 he was already spending money on the drug,[65] and three years later he sold books and medical instruments to satisfy the cravings which had already become insatiable.[66] Because of the habit, in 1887 he lost a job given him by a kindly shoemaker.[67] Twelve years later the elder Meynell induced him to go to a private hospital for cure.[68] Although the impression left by the biography is that this treatment succeeded, a later record indicates that its success must have been temporary at best; for in November, 1907, Thompson confessed to Wilfrid Meynell, "I am dying from laudanum poisoning." [69]

That Thompson experienced, too, the usual opium dreams, is certain. Thus, Meynell comments, "his letters contain complaints of dreams akin to Coleridge's," and then quotes Thompson's description of "a most miserable fortnight of torpid, despondent days, and affrightful nights, dreams having been in part the worst realities of my life." [70]

I have not space to deal in detail with Thompson's poetry, although much of it is swiftly phantasmagoric, often approaching the imagery we have come to recognize as a consequence of addiction to opium. The danger is that one may go too far and attribute, glibly, all its strangeness to a "ghostly aura from quick-burning nerves." [71] Thompson himself has tempted such overemphasis by the following testament in a poem suggestively entitled "The Poppy":

THE MILK OF PARADISE

> The sleep-flower sways in the wheat its head,
> Heavy with dreams, as that with bread. . . .
>
> I hang 'mid men my needless head,
> And my fruit is dreams, as theirs is bread. . . .
>
> Love! *I* fall into the claws of Time:
> But lasts within a leavèd rhyme
> All that the world of me esteems —
> My withered dreams, my withered dreams.[72]

Thompson's work also includes a prose fantasy, "Finis Coronat Opus," closely comparable to DeQuincey's visions of pain. Again, as in "Sir Eustace," the opium vagaries are moulded to fit a narrative frame designed to account for them, and again the pretext for the persecution is a murder; for the poet Florentian buys genius from an evil spirit at the price of killing his own sweetheart. Perhaps because of Thompson's inherent sensitivity, light phenomena are stressed early in the story. He describes a multitude of parti-colored lamps:

> Above them were coiled thinnest serpentinings of suspended crystal, hued like the tongues in a wintry hearth, flame-colour, violet, and green; so that, as in the heated current from the lamps the snakes twirled and flickered and their bright shadows twirled upon the wall, they seemed at length to undulate their twines, and the whole

altar became surmounted with a fiery fantasy of sinuous stains.[73]

These sinuous undulations of light rays on a narcotized retina are very like the experiences of Sir Eustace.[74]

Dupouy treats at some length the effect of opium on auditory perceptions, of which some signs have already appeared in De-Quincey and Crabbe:

> L'ouïe devient d'une délicatesse exquise; les moindres bruits sont perçus . . . la marche d'un insecte sur le sol . . . le froissement d'une herbe . . . et si ce bruit revêt une intensité tant soit peu marquée, l'oreille est douloureusement affectée.[75]

The contrasted blasting and exquisiteness of sound effects, so difficult to describe in terms of normal audition, occur within a single paragraph of "Finis Coronat Opus"; for with hearing as with sight, there is no quiescence in the opium world; everything is in a constant flux of intensification or recession. To Florentian appears an idol, "soaked with fire."

> There issued from the lips a voice that threw Florentian on the ground: "Whom seekest thou?" . . . A voice came forth again, but a voice that sounded not the same; a voice that seemed to

have withered in crossing the confines of existence, and to traverse illimitable remotenesses beyond the imagining of man; a voice melancholy with a boundless calm, the calm not of a crystalline peace but of a marmoreal despair, "Knowest thou me; who I am?" [76]

Later is repeated the effect of attenuated sound on ear drums almost painfully keen. With it appears the familiar persecution theme, again through time without end, but in a new form: the hypnotic effect of accusing eyes holds the dreamer as a snake's stare holds a bird.[77] The poet strikes down his bride, and

then — her eyes opened. I *saw* them open, through the gloom I saw them; through the gloom they were revealed to me, that I might see them to my hour of death.... Motionless with horror they were fixed on mine, motionless with horror mine were fixed on them, as she wakened into death.

How long had I seen them? I saw them still. ... All my senses are resolved into one sense, and that is frozen to those eyes. Silence now, at least, abysmal silence; except the sound (or is the sound in me?), the sound of dripping blood, except that the flame upon the altar sputters, and hisses, and bickers, as if it licked its jaws. Yes! there is another sound — hush, hark! It is the throbbing of my heart.... The loud pulse dies slowly away ... and again I hear the licking of the flame.[78]

A flash again of undulating light phenomena, as he sees that "the hideous, green, writhing tongue was streaked and flaked with *red*! I swooned . . . swooned to myself, but swooned not to those eyes." [79]

A monstrosity appears, like the crocodile which had kissed DeQuincey "with cancerous kisses": "When I recovered consciousness, it was risen from the ground, and kissed me with the kisses of its mouth." [80] And the persecution goes on and on, sustained by an agency as persistent as the "fiends" we already know. "For two years . . . it had spoken to me with her lips, used her gestures, smiled her smile."[81] And long afterward:

> I can fly no farther, I fall exhausted, the fanged hour fastens on my throat . . . hurrying retributions whose multitudinous tramplings converge upon me in a hundred presages, in a hundred shrivelling menaces, down all the echoing avenues of doom.[82]

Although Coleridge, who had taken opium several times before 1791, was the first author of the four to experience the effects of the drug,[83] I have hitherto reserved treatment of his work, in order to gain all possible

[27]

THE MILK OF PARADISE

momentum of evidence before approaching the contested question: did opium influence the composition of "The Ancient Mariner"? The problem hinges upon the issue whether before the conception of the poem in November, 1797, Coleridge had experienced the type of opium dreams which might have exerted such influence.

The data concerning Coleridge's early use of opium I have collected in an appendix. The indubitable facts are: one, that as early as 1791 Coleridge had tried opium; and two, that the suffering which led him to do so continued until 1796, when definite proofs of addiction occur in March, and again in November and December. An investigation of the works which he composed in 1796 reveals, too, startling indications that he had experienced, even in that year, not only the pleasures, but the pains attendant either upon long addiction or upon overdoses.

In Coleridge's Note Book of random jottings, upon which Professor Lowes has based his study of Coleridge's reading,[84] occurs a series of passages about which, Mr. Lowes confesses, except for some possible resemblances to a lightning storm in Bartram's

Travels, he has "not the remotest notion what they are." [85] The following quotation is a part of "one of the most wildly incoherent pages of the Note Book," [86] spaced just as Coleridge jotted it:

> a dusky light — a purple *flash*
> crystalline splendor — light blue —
>   *Green* lightnings —
> in that eternal and delirious (misery) [87]
>   wrath fires —
>   inward desolations
>   an horror of great darkness
>   great things — on the ocean
>   counterfeit infinity — [88]

The time of the three pages of these confused entries [89] has been definitely placed in the month or two before the composition of the "Ode to the Departing Year," written December 24–26, 1796. Upon this point, based on the inclusion of germinating fragments of the "Ode" amid the entries, Campbell,[90] Lowes,[91] and Brandl [92] unhesitatingly agree. The significant thing is that in Coleridge's letters of those months, we discover more frequent references to his recourse to opium than he ever made again within the same length of time.[93]

It is fairly clear that the disorder of these

pages is due to extravagances induced by a combination of drugs and physical pain, and that at least the passage I have quoted is an excerpt from an opium vision itself. The hitherto inexplicable confusion of entries is shot through, moreover, with indications that Coleridge was preoccupied at that period with the subjects of opium and dreams. In the Note Book, immediately preceding the first fragment of the "Ode to the Departing Year," is the statement: "Dreams sometimes useful by giving to the well-grounded fears and hopes of the understanding the feelings of vivid sense." [94] Immediately following the same fragment occurs what is evidently Coleridge's description of a dream of pain: "In a distempered dream things and forms in themselves common and harmless inflict a terror of anguish"; [95] and this statement is in turn followed by another bit from the "Ode." [96] Farther on, in the first draft of a scene later used in *Osorio*, occurs a mysterious reference to opium:

> It had been a damning sin to have remained
> An opium chewer with such excellent grapes
> Over his cottage.[97]

THE MILK OF PARADISE

And finally, on the same incoherent page with the "green lightnings" passage, come significant jottings of "deep sighings," and "unbind the poppy garland," which again may possibly be allusions to opium.

Even without these vanes to point the wind, internal evidence indicates the opium origin of the excerpt I quoted above. The lights and colors are certainly as close to Crabbe's "dancing streamers" and Thomson's color experiences of red, violet, and green crystal as they are to Bartram's lightnings. The rest of the passage, which an appeal to Bartram leaves entirely unexplained, is paralleled in every detail by known opium phenomena. The "eternal and delirious misery," the "wrath fires," "desolations," and "horror" represent again that omnipresent theme of persecution through eternity; and in the "great things" and "counterfeit infinity" of the ocean, space once more undergoes its limitless expansion.

In the "Ode to the Departing Year" itself — a poem in which, as Brandl puts it, Coleridge's "Gemütserregung steigert sich bis ins Fieberhafte" [98] — are evidences of opium delirium even more definite than the confusion of the structure. In one passage Coleridge describes a horrible vision which has appeared to him:

> And ever, when the dream of night
> Renews the phantom to my sight,
> Cold sweat-drops gather on my limbs;
> My ears throb hot; my eye-balls start,
> My brain with horrid tumult swims;
> Wild is the tempest of my heart;
> And my thick and struggling breath
> Imitates the toil of death!

If there is doubt that these lines refer to the effects of a dream of terror caused by opium,[99] a striking parallel occurs in "The Pains of Sleep," 1803,[100] which Coleridge himself classifies with the opium dream, "Kubla Khan." [101] Its similarities both to DeQuincey's experiences and to the excerpt above are apparent even from a few lines of quotation:

> But yester-night I prayed aloud
> In anguish and in agony,
> Up-starting from the fiendish crowd
> Of shapes and thoughts that tortured me:
> A lurid light, a trampling throng,
> Sense of intolerable wrong,
> And whom I scorned, those only strong! . . .

THE MILK OF PARADISE

> Desire with loathing strangely mixed
> On wild or hateful objects fixed. . . .

> For all seemed guilt, remorse or woe.

And farther on in the same poem, he describes

> The third night, when my own loud scream
> Had waked me from the fiendish dream.

Such dreams in 1803, when Coleridge was undeniably deep in the toils of opium, are understandable; but, in view of the traditional opinion, it may still be hard to believe that the dreams also occurred as early as the "Ode" of December, 1796. A letter of Coleridge's dated September 22, 1803, clinches the case. After relating the same dreams described in the "Pains of Sleep," from which, awakening, he "blest the scream which delivered him from reluctant sleep," he makes this neglected statement: "Nine years ago I had three months' visitation of this kind." [102] "Nine years ago" would have been in 1794. Certainly there is no reason here for conscious misstatement, and even Coleridge's fickle memory could not have recalled as "nine years" anything less than seven years. It seems probable that Coleridge is remem-

THE MILK OF PARADISE

bering, although hazily in regard to date, the very dreams of 1796 with which we are concerned.[103]

In the afternoon of November 13, 1797, Coleridge conceived the plan of "The Ancient Mariner," and brought the poem, completed, to read to the Wordsworths on the evening of March 23, 1798.[104] Now that we know Coleridge had already experienced opium dreams of horror in 1796 of sufficient intensity to have left their impress on his poems of that year, the question of the influence of opium on "The Ancient Mariner" must be viewed in a new light. The problem resolves itself into two distinct questions: whether opium had a part in inspiring the conception and scheme of the work; and aside from that, whether the scenery and sensations of Coleridge's dreams were utilized in the details of the poem.

Mr. John Mackinnon Robertson, in the answer to the first question which has had so much influence on the popular conception of Coleridge, represents the type of criticism I am trying to avoid. At one fell swoop he stigmatizes "The Ancient Mariner," the first part of "Christabel," and "Kubla

Khan" as "an abnormal product of an abnormal nature under abnormal conditions," [105] all having been "conceived and composed under the influence of opium." [106]

In view of the phantasmagoric quality of all drug visions, I concur with Mr. Lowes in his denial of the specious theory that so highly wrought a piece of conscious artistry as "The Ancient Mariner" could have been "*composed* under the influence of opium," [107] but I cannot agree with him that opium played no part in the inspiration of the poem.

There can be no question of the great gulf, both in subject and style, between "The Ancient Mariner" and Coleridge's earlier work, which had tended to didacticism and rhetoric, and had employed, in Coleridge's own scornful words, "such shadowy nobodies as cherub-winged *Death*, Trees of *Hope*, bare-bosomed *Affection* and simpering *Peace*." [108] Reduced to baldest terms, the factors to which Mr. Lowes attributes this change are the influence of William and Dorothy Wordsworth, and "that equipoise of the intellectual and emotional faculties, which [Coleridge] christened 'joy!'" [109]

These causes explain a gradual ripening

rather than a sudden metamorphosis of technique, and leave unexplained Coleridge's use of the supernatural theme so foreign to Wordsworth's temperament. I put most of my faith in Mr. Lowes's final hypothesis:

> Above all, for the first time in his life Coleridge had hit upon a theme which fired his imagination, and set him voyaging again through all the wonder-haunted regions of all his best-loved books.[110]

The point where I differ from Mr. Lowes is in my belief that this theme was not a happy accident of the imagination, but had its source and development in Coleridge's opium hallucinations. We have seen that such dreams had already influenced Coleridge's poetry, and might be very likely do so again. Against this theory, too, the objection that the "superb, unwavering imaginative control" of the poem "is not the gift of opium"[111] would not be valid. "The Ancient Mariner," I venture to say, underwent the same process to which both "Sir Eustace Grey" and "Finis Coronat Opus" were subjected: a framework of plot was constructed expressly to contain the pre-existent fabric of dream phenomena.

A careful interpretation of Wordsworth's account of the poem's origin bears out this theory. In the course of a walk, he says,

> was planned the poem of the "Ancient Mariner," founded on a dream, as Mr. Coleridge said, of his friend Mr. Cruikshank. Much the greatest part of the story was Mr. Coleridge's invention; but certain parts I suggested; for example, some crime was to be committed which should bring upon the Old Navigator . . . the spectral persecution.[112]

Wordsworth also related to the Reverend Alexander Dyce substantially the same story of the famous walk, with the additional detail that the original dream was of "a skeleton ship, with figures in it." [113] Wordsworth's accounts agree that his own share in the poem was limited to the suggestion of two incidents: the shooting of the albatross, and the navigation of the ship by the dead men.

The significant information here is to be read between the lines. Coleridge seized upon the detail of "a skeleton ship," but the spectral persecution is his own idea. Wordsworth evidently added, after its conception, the detail of a crime to motivate this persecution. And by the time Wordsworth later suggested the supernatural navigation, it is apparent that the plot had been completed, up to this point, by Coleridge himself.

DeQuincey, moreover, gives evidence that such a plan had been forming in Coleridge's mind, independently of Cruikshanks's dream:

> It is very possible, from something which Coleridge said on another occasion, that, before meeting a fable in which to embody his ideas, he had meditated a poem on delirium, confounding its own dream-scenery with external things, and connected with the imagery of high latitudes.[114]

And this account, Mr. Lowes affirms, "carries its own conviction." [115]

"A poem on delirium," "dream scenery," "spectral persecution"! These compose the structure which rose at once in Coleridge's mind at the mere suggestion of a skeleton ship. Finally, notice DeQuincey's statement that this material *preceded* the conception of "a fable in which to embody his ideas." What better confirmation could there be not only of the hypothesis that the inspiration of "The Ancient Mariner" was an opium dream of persecution, but also that the plot was a consciously designed framework of later addition?

THE MILK OF PARADISE

The effect of opium on the poetry of George Crabbe has already been discussed. His imagination, too, was unleashed from his desire to portray humble life "as Truth will paint it," [116] and went soaring into the "high latitudes" [117] with their fiends, and horrors, and spectral persecutions. But he returned at once to rustic subjects and a lukewarm style. For Coleridge, the dreams sent his creative imagination voyaging in the strange literature of Elizabethan travellers and alchemistic handbooks, which harmonized so well with his dream experiences; and all these elements, fused in the heat of his imagination, were later consciously shaped into the artistic whole which is "The Ancient Mariner." [118]

The possibility of opium influences on the details of the poem is not eliminated by the fact that Mr. Lowes has already traced much of the imagery of "The Ancient Mariner" to parallels in Coleridge's reading. Opium dreams, as DeQuincey indicates, feed upon the fragmentary memories of earlier experience.[119] From the Note Book it is evident that Coleridge had opium hallucinations while in the very process of reading about the

THE MILK OF PARADISE

material he later utilized in the poem. It is almost unbelievable that scenes which impressed him so vividly should not sink into his memory, to be later metamorphosed in the crucible of dreams; [120] and indeed, as Mr. Lowes points out, this is the actual process recorded in "Kubla Khan"![121] Possibly, too, Coleridge more or less consciously clothed the bits from his reading in the new and glowing material of his dream memories. Whatever the explanation, this is a matter incapable of absolute proof. It is for me but to present parallels; the decision must be left to the reader.

Sir Eustace had murdered a friend; Florentian had slain his sweetheart; the Ancient Mariner had killed an albatross. It is the killing of the albatross which sets off the long train of "spectral persecution."[122] As Sir Eustace had attributed his sufferings to the "two fiends of darkness," Florentian to an indescribable monster, DeQuincey to a Malay, so the Mariner places all the blame on a spirit. And significantly, some of the sailors "*in dreams* assured were" of the fiend who had engineered all the persecution. Throughout the endless duration of these tortures (no track is kept of time, but the general impression is of interminable extension) appear other characteristic phenomena.

The equivalent of DeQuincey's "unutterable abortions" occur in

> The very deep did rot: O Christ! ...
>
> Yea, slimy things did crawl with legs
> Upon the slimy sea. ...
>
> And a thousand thousand slimy things
> Lived on; and so did I.

And again in

> I looked upon the rotting sea.

There are, too, frequent reminiscences of the terrors of sleep:

> Fear at my heart, as at a cup,
> My life-blood seemed to sip.

And once occurs almost the very wording of the dream in the "Ode to the Departing Year," with its "my ears throb hot, my eye balls start," and the "cold sweat drops" that "gather on my limbs":

> I closed my lids, and kept them close,
> And the balls like pulses beat;

THE MILK OF PARADISE

> For the sky and the sea, and the sea and the sky
> Lay like a load on my weary eye.

And later:

> The cold sweat melted from their limbs.

Perhaps the most striking descriptions are those of light and color. Remembering the serpentining mass of "flame-colour, violet, and green" in "Finis Coronat Opus," can we attribute Coleridge's perceptions to a different source? [123]

> About, about, in reel and rout
> The death fires danced at night;
> The water like a witch's oils
> Burnt green, and blue, and white.

The same picture of writhing snakes which Thompson used to express this sinuous motion is repeated by Coleridge:

> They moved in tracks of shining white,
> And when they reared, the elfish light
> Fell off in hoary flakes. ...

> Blue, glassy green, and velvet black,
> They coiled and swam; and every track
> Was a flash of golden fire.

The "dancing streamers" of Sir Eustace's visions play again in the Mariner's sky, in a passage of sound, movement, even wording amazingly close to that of Crabbe:

> The upper air burst into life!
> And a hundred fire-flags sheen.
> To and fro they were hurried about!
> And to and fro, and in and out,
> The wan stars danced between.

Later the effect is repeated:

> Like waters shot from some high crag,
> The lightning fell with never a jag,
> A river steep and wide.

Sound perception again ranges between the two extremes upon which Dupouy has commented. There is the crash of noise on abnormally sensitive ear drums:

> It cracked and growled, and roared and howled,
> Like noises in a swound! . . .
>
> The ice did split with a thunder-fit.

And at the end of the poem, sound becomes loud enough to sink the ship! But there is also the "délicatesse exquise" of hearing:

> With far-heard whisper, o'er the sea,
> Off shot the spectre-bark. . . .
>
> And every soul, it passed me by,
> Like the whiz of my cross-bow.[124]

Yet another similarity in a detail of persecution is "the curse of the eye" which played so prominent a part in "Finis Coronat Opus." I can only summarize the Mariner's frequent references to this appearance. The first is:

> Each turned his face with a ghastly pang,
> And cursed me with his eye.

This look, we discover, "had never passed away," and was seen "seven days and seven nights"; later their "stony eyes" again gleamed in the moon; still, he "could not draw his eyes from theirs"; and finally,

> Their stony eye-balls glitter'd on
> In the red and smoky light.[125]

Even from the quotations given, although they contain the more obvious similarities only, can be seen how significantly close is the imagery of "The Ancient Mariner" to the opium effects we already know. Such parallels can be extended, less certainly, to most of the details of the poem: for example, thirsty "Death" and "Life in Death" and the sensation of floating.[126]

To its quotation by Mr. Lowes [127] I owe the original draft of another poem which seems clearly the product of opium, despite the obscurity of this fact in its later and familiar version.[128] It was found in a note book dated 1800, prefaced by Coleridge's own hastily jotted note: [129]

> It is eleven o'clock at night. See that conical volcano of coal, half-an-inch high, ejaculating its inverted cone of smoke — the smoke in what a furious mood — this way, that way, and what a noise!

Not only is the flection of the smoke typical of opium perceptions, but Coleridge's extreme sensitivity to the noise of the burning coal is exactly like Florentian's perception of the loudly bickering flame in "Finis Coronat Opus." The poem itself is even more revealing, with the felicitous expression of that sublime expansion of space which opium effects:

> The poet's eye in his tipsy hour [130]
> Hath a magnifying power,
> Or rather emancipates his eyes
> Of the accidents of size.
> In unctuous cone of kindling coal,
> Or smoke from his pipe's bole,
>   His eye can see
>   Phantoms of sublimity.

With "Kubla Khan" we reach the end of this little pilgrimage through "straunge

THE MILK OF PARADISE

strondes." This poem does not merely reconstruct the world of dreams; it was itself composed within that very land. Coleridge's account of its composition is too familiar to need repetition in full. Enough that in the summer of 1798,[131] under influence of an "anodyne" now definitely known to have been opium,[132] he fell asleep while reading in *Purchas his Pilgrimage*, and in that state composed a poem "in which all the images rose up before him as *things*, with a parallel production of the correspondent expressions without any sensation or consciousness of effort." [133] The recording of this dream composition upon awakening was interrupted at the fifty-fourth line, and was never completed.[134]

Thus Coleridge's verse caught up the evanescent images of an opium dream, and struck them into immobility for all time. The dream quality of "Kubla Khan" cannot be analyzed; like the rainbow tints of a butterfly's wing, it turns to dust on the fingers. But the swift shuttling of vistas is there to perfection. From "Alph, the sacred river" the scene shifts to brilliant gardens; then, after a flash of "that deep romantic

THE MILK OF PARADISE

chasm," turns to the dome of pleasure; and suddenly, in that vision within a vision, emerge the glowing forms of the "Abyssinian maid" with a dulcimer, and the wild-haired youth who, like Coleridge, has "drunk the milk of Paradise." [135]

No pain phenomena occur in the poem, for this is that rarity, a dream of pleasure purely, with all the intoxication and none of the tortures of opium. But Mr. Lowes's quick eye has caught, as most characteristic of "Kubla Khan," an effect which we know is the mark of opium: the extraordinary mutations of space. The little river at the opening of the poem expands into a mighty fountain which flings rocks like chaff; contracts into a peacefully meandering creek; then, by another dilation, becomes a huge primordial river sinking through measureless caverns — and all at once is the pellucid stream of the sunny dome of pleasure.[136] And through all is maintained a restless ebb and flow of style, to match the eternal unrest of the dream scenery itself.

The Mrs. Barbaulds are always with us, although the criticism of the early nineteenth century that "The Ancient Mariner" "had no moral"[137] now gives place to the more sophisticated demand that the entire poem be discarded as the product of a pathological mentality.[138] But surely the Mrs. Barbaulds are wrong. The important fact is that these four authors did an incredible thing: they opened to poetry an entirely new world. And with Coleridge and the apotheosis of this poetry in "Kubla Khan" came that rarest phenomenon, the true originality which is not just the "repristination of something old,"[139] but is something no one had conceived since poetry began. With it was struck that "new note" of lyricism[140] of which the reverberations have not yet died away.

Alas! the vision and the flight are pitifully brief before outraged nature exacts its vengeance. For "opium gives and takes away," as DeQuincey said,[141] and while aspirations and projects are exalted, the will to execute is soon blasted.[142] Pathetic footnotes in the annals of literature are the tremendous metaphysical tractates both Coleridge and DeQuincey planned, but neither ever began.[143] In Shelley's figure, "the mind in creation is as a fading coal," and although the wind of opium may fan it into an instant's supernal brightness, the flame soon exhausts its fuel, wavers, and dies.

For fleeting moments of relief and revelation, Coleridge paid with a loss of creative power,[144] even of moral sense,[145] and with a lifetime of physical and mental torture. But to those moments we owe part of "The Ancient Mariner," all of "Kubla Khan," and both are like oases in our dusty lives. There is nothing frightening in their rich strangeness. Rather, they are to be the more dearly cherished because of the fearful toll exacted for beauty stolen from another world.

APPENDIX

APPENDIX

Coleridge's Use of Opium before 1798

THE earliest evidence of Coleridge's use of opium occurs in a letter to his brother George, dated November 28, 1791, in which Coleridge describes a painful attack of rheumatism, and then suddenly remarks: "Opium never used to have any disagreeable effects on me — but it has on many." [1] That Coleridge, even at nineteen, could speak familiarly of past indulgences in the drug, and the evident association in his mind between rheumatism and opium, makes it probable that Professor Lowes is right when he states, "there is every reason to believe . . . that laudanum had been prescribed for [Coleridge] at school (which he had left but two months before), when he was suffering from rheumatic fever." [2]

The implications go even farther. For every sort of pain opium, we know, was freely prescribed, even for children, by doctors of the late eighteenth century.[3] And there is much evidence that Coleridge as a boy was uncommonly subject to physical distresses. In a letter to Poole, October 16, 1797, Coleridge describes how he had run away, when a child of seven, to avoid punishment for a serious fault, and how he had been exposed to a rain storm all through a cold October night. When found, he says, "I was put to bed and recovered in a day or so, but I was certainly injured. For I was weakly and subject to the ague for many years after." [4] Campbell records another such adventure, which befell Coleridge as a schoolboy:

> Once, as he told Gillman (Gillman's Life, p. 33), he swam across the New River in his clothes, and let them dry on his back, with the consequence, apparently, that "full half his time from seventeen to eighteen was passed in the sick-ward of Christ's hospital, afflicted with jaundice and rheumatic fever." [5]

In the summer of 1790, Coleridge himself, in a "Sonnet on Pain," speaks of "frequent pangs," and the "Seas of Pain" which "seem waving through each limb." [6]

At any rate it is certain that before 1791, and in that year, Coleridge was taking opium for rheumatic pain. As there are frequent indications that this subjection to pain and illness continued, it is probable that the use of

APPENDIX

opium for relief continued as well. Thus, Campbell mentions a letter of 1792 in which Coleridge complains of toothache;[7] and in other letters of February 5, 1793,[8] and of February 9, 1793,[9] Coleridge complains again of a decayed tooth, and consequent fever. On April 12, 1794, he also describes a "violent pain in his limbs," which almost prevents him from writing.[10]

On Saturday, March 12, 1796, Coleridge wrote to the Reverend Mr. Edwards:

> Since I last wrote you, I have been tottering on the verge of madness — my mind overbalanced on the *e contra* side of happiness — the blunders of my associate, etc., etc., abroad, and, at home, Mrs. Coleridge dangerously ill. . . . Such has been my situation for the last fortnight — I have been obliged to take laudanum almost every night.[11]

That this turmoil of mind dates back at least to February 22 is evident in a letter of that date,[12] and that it lasted until the end of March is clear from a letter to Poole of March 30.[13] The significant point here is that now Coleridge is taking opium, for a few weeks at least, not for pain, but for mental troubles. This, as Hahn points out, is the indication of danger.[14] I disagree, then, with

THE MILK OF PARADISE

Mr. Lowes that "the first hint of the deadly peril lurking in the remedy appears in the letter of April, 1798 [15] . . . for in the reference to the divine repose of opium and to the spot of enchantment which it creates a new and ominous note is heard." [16] The ominous note had in reality sounded two years before that date.

The greatest siege of the drug came in the last two months of 1796. On Saturday night, November 5, Coleridge wrote to Poole:

> On Wednesday night I was seized with an intolerable pain from my right temple to the tip of my right shoulder, including my right eye, cheek, jaw, and that side of the throat. . . . It came on . . . several times on Thursday . . . but I took between sixty and seventy drops of laudanum, and sopped the cerberus. . . . But this morning he returned in full force, and his name is Legion. . . . I have a blister under my right ear, and I take twenty-five drops of laudanum every five hours, the ease and *spirits* gained by which have enabled me to write you this flighty but not exaggerated account.[17]

For several days, then, it is certain that Coleridge took opium in large amounts. Mr. Lowes has added another bit of evidence by his quotation of Coleridge's unpublished note to Cottle, evidently referring to the same

APPENDIX

occasion. "I have a blister under my right ear — and I take laudanum every few hours, twenty-five drops each dose." [18] Cottle added a postscript to the hastily scrawled note: "Oh that S. T. C. had never taken more than twenty-five drops each dose." [19]

On December 13, 1796, Coleridge wrote a wildly confused letter to Poole, about which Campbell says:

It is a whirl of appeals, adjurations, reproaches, cries *de profundis*, plans and plans of life framed and torn up and resumed to be again abandoned, in bewildering profusion.[20]

In view of the evidence of the recourse to opium the month before, and the "flighty" letter which resulted, it seems clear that this second letter to Poole had a like origin.

There is evidence that the painful afflictions of November continued through the next month. On December 17, 1796, Coleridge describes another "rheumatic pain in the back of my head and shoulders, accompanied with sore throat and depression of the animal spirits"; [21] and on the next day, in a letter to Poole, we get a further account:

I am very poorly, not to say ill. My face monstrously swollen — my recondite eye sits distent quaintly . . . and I have a sore throat that prevents my eating aught but spoon-meat without great pain. And I have a rheumatic complaint in the back part of my head and shoulders![22]

And on December 26, in the dedication of the "Ode to the Departing Year," Coleridge refers again to the rheumatic complaint as having lasted until December 24.[23] His painful ailments, some recourse to opium, and the probability of continued addiction thus extended through both months.

There is later indirect evidence which may also point to continued, although irregular, use of opium before the composition of "The Ancient Mariner." Coleridge writes to Joseph Cottle in the spring of 1797:

> On the Saturday, the Sunday, and the ten days after my arrival at Stowey, I felt a depression too dreadful to be described. . . . I am not the man I have been — and I think I never shall; a sort of calm hopelessness diffuses itself over my heart.[24]

When we realize that in March he had already taken opium to relieve such mental strain, the following statement to Thelwall is ominous:

> I should much wish, like the Indian Vishnu, to float about along an infinite ocean cradled in the

APPENDIX

flower of the Lotus, and wake once in a million years more.[25]

And in April, 1798, comes this letter to his brother:

> Laudanum gave me repose, not sleep: but you, I believe, know how divine that repose is, what a spot of enchantment, a green spot of fountain and flowers and trees in the very heart of a waste of sands.[26]

This was written just after the completion of "The Ancient Mariner," but the significance is in the note of *reminiscence* of the pleasures found in opium. It was in the very next month, May, 1798, that "as a result of a serious quarrel with Lloyd," Coleridge took the opium dose which resulted in "Kubla Khan."

From this material it is evident that Coleridge had taken opium to assuage pain at least several times before 1791, and that he probably continued to do so for the painful afflictions which came in succeeding years. On March 12, 1796, he took opium "almost every night" for mental disturbances which had already lasted a fortnight, and which continued until the end of the month. We know definitely that in November of the

THE MILK OF PARADISE

same year, on Thursday the third, he took opium, and that on the following Saturday, at four or five hour intervals, he took large doses. This time the painful condition lasted for two months, until December 26. Certainly it is not rash to assume that the recourse to opium continued as well. In the spring of 1797, Coleridge again felt the great depression of mind which had already led to opium in the past; and in March comes the significant reference to opium as a "spot of enchantment."

At all events, it is certain that Coleridge, before the conception of "The Ancient Mariner," had sufficiently experienced the effects of opium to make the proof of its influence on "The Ancient Mariner" dependent only upon evidence in the poem itself.[27]

NOTES

NOTES

1. *The Odyssey*, Butcher and Lang translation, book IV. There seems no doubt that Homer refers to opium. See Louis Lewin, *Phantastica*, London, 1931, p. 34; Benno Hahn, *Die Morphin-Erkrangungen*, Heidelberg, 1927, pp. 1-2; Charles E. Terry and Mildred Peelens, *The Opium Problem*, New York, 1928, p. 55.
2. *Georgics*, I, 78. "Lethaeo perfusa papavero somno."
3. *Aeneid*, IV, 486. "Spargens humida melle soporiferumque papaver."
4. *Complete Works of Geoffrey Chaucer*, ed. F. N. Robinson, New York, 1933; "The Knight's Tale," ll. 1471-1472; "The Legend of Good Women," ll. 2669-2670.
5. *Othello*, III, iii, 331.
6. *Comus*, ll. 675-676.
7. *Letters of Samuel Taylor Coleridge*, ed. Ernest Hartley Coleridge, London, 1895, I, 240.
8. *The Collected Writings of Thomas DeQuincey*, ed. David Masson, London, 1896, III, 395.
9. Arthur Symons, "The Opium Smoker," *Days and Nights*, London and New York, 1889, p. 18.
10. Roger Dupouy, *Les Opiomanes*, Paris, 1912, p. 93.
11. "Suspiria de Profundis," *Writings*, XIII, 339.
12. *Ibid.*, p. 335.

THE MILK OF PARADISE

13. *Life of Francis Thompson*, New York, 1926.
14. *Life of the Rev. George Crabbe*, Cambridge and Boston, 1834.
15. See p. 14, below.
16. *Selections from DeQuincey*, ed. M. H. Turk (*Athenaeum Press Series*), Boston, 1902, p. 151. This edition contains the first and shorter version of the *Confessions*.
17. "Recollections of Charles Lamb," *Writings*, III, 76; Letter in *London Magazine*, *Writings*, III, 464–465.
18. "Confessions," *Writings*, III, 379. (This is the revised and longer version of 1856.)
19. To understand why authors from DeQuincey to Thompson were so easily induced to take opium, it must be realized that medical opinion from the time of Hippocrates and Galen until well on in the nineteenth century concurred in praise of the drug as "a sacred anchor of life." As late as 1791, a certain Hast Handy recommended opium for all diseases from dyspepsia to syphilis, and added a gratuitous encomium on "the charm of this agreeable ecstasy." (Terry, *The Opium Habit*, pp. 59–60.) See also Lewin, *Phantastica*, pp. 37–41.
20. "Confessions," *Athenaeum Edition*, p. 157.
21. See Dupouy's distinction between "la reverie" of early addiction, with its pleasant processions of idealized scenery, and "l'intoxication et l'ivresse," which proceed from an overdose or from long continued addiction, and in which the hallucinations become disordered, terrifying, and more vividly realistic.

NOTES

22. David Masson, *DeQuincey*, London, 1926; *Writings*, XIII, 337.
23. The period of DeQuincey's addiction and his spasmodic attempts at abstinence, so obscure in his accounts, is summed up in the *Athenaeum Edition*, p. 468. Although re-worked opium dreams occur in "Suspiria de Profundis," "Daughter of Lebanon," and "The English Mail Coach" (*Athenaeum Edition*, pp. 470–471), they repeat the phenomena of the *Confessions*.
24. "Confessions," *Writings*, III, 434.
25. London, 1926, p. 28.
26. *Les Opiomanes*, pp. 99–100. The same effect is cited by D. W. Cheever, "Narcotics," *North American Review*, XCV (1862), 388.
27. "Confessions," *Writings*, III, 435.
28. *Les Opiomanes*, p. 100.
29. *Ibid.*, p. 115. Confirmation of these symptoms occurs in almost any opium chronicle. See Cheever, *North American Review*, XCV (1862), 388; Walter Cotton, *Knickerbocker Magazine*, VII (1836), 421. Baudelaire, the French opium poet, testifies in "Le Poison" (*Oeuvres Complètes de Charles Baudelaire*, Paris, 1922, *Les Fleurs du Mal*, p. 80):

> L'opium aggrandit ce qui n'a pas de bornes,
> Allonge l'illimité,
> Approfondit le temps.

That Arthur Symons has written an opium poem will surprise many. His sonnet, "The Opium Smoker" (*Days and Nights*, London, 1889, p. 18), is so little known, yet so clearly describes the same twisted sense perceptions in a rare vision of pleasure, that the octave is worth quoting in full. The italics are mine:

> I am engulfed, and drown deliciously.
> Soft music like a perfume, and sweet light
> Golden with audible odors exquisite,
> Swathe me with cerements *for eternity*.
> *Time is no more.* I pause and yet I flee.
> *A million ages* wrap me round with night.
> I drain *a million ages* of delight.
> I hold the future in my memory.

30. "Confessions," *Writings*, pp. 439–441. Bodies of water seem characteristic of much dream scenery. (See Baudelaire, *Petits Poèmes en Prose*, Paris, 1869.) Ludlow, again, describes similar visions from hasheesh (*The Hasheesh Eater*, p. 34).
31. "Confessions," *Writings*, III, 440.
32. *Ibid.*, pp. 402–405.
33. *Ibid.*, pp. 441–442.
34. *Ibid.*, p. 443. Italics mine.
35. *Ibid.* These monstrous appearances suggest a phase of addiction to opium that modern psychology seems to neglect. Opium may be eaten, smoked, injected subcutaneously as morphine, or drunk in the form of laudanum (Dupouy, p. 22). In each case, the effects differ widely. (See Jean Cocteau, *Opium*, New York, 1932, pp. 94–95.) DeQuincey, in the period of these visions, drank 8,000 drops of laudanum each day (*Writings*, p. 401). Since laudanum is opium dissolved in alcohol, he consumed at the same time 48 ounces of proof spirits, composed, in turn, of 50% to 60% grain alcohol (John W. Robertson,

NOTES

Edgar A. Poe, New York, 1923, pp. 65–66).
DeQuincy drank, then, the equivalent of a
pint of whiskey each day. Since Dupouy
maintains that the ordinary opium vision is
pleasant (pp. 107, 173) — although he mentions experiences similar to DeQuincey's following excessive indulgences in opium alone
— the dreams of "physical horror," as opposed to the "moral and spiritual terror,"
may very well be due to this attendant
alcoholic indulgence. Such an assumption
seems to be confirmed by the description of
alcohol hallucinations of "monsters, serpents
. . . vermin, reptiles . . . monkeys," etc.
(Edmund Parish, *Hallucinations and Illusions*, London, 1897, pp. 41–43. *Cf.* George B.
Cutten, *The Psychology of Alcoholism*, New
York, 1907, pp. 148–149).

36. *Confessions of an English Opium-Eater*, ed.
Richard Garnett, London, 1885, p. 263.
37. *Ibid.*, pp. 263–264.
38. *Writings*, III, 444–445.
39. *Ibid.*, p. 446.
40. *Ibid.*, pp. 446–447. A few opium users deny
that the drug is conducive to visions at all.
(See the anonymous *Opium Habit*, New York,
1868, p. 53; Robertson, *Poe*, p. 67.) The evidence of DeQuincey, the long and scholarly
analysis of opium visions, based on numerous
observations, by Dupouy in *Les Opiomanes*,
and the testimony of other addicts whom I
quote throughout the essay, is surely enough
to refute such a belief. But this conflict of
testimony can easily be reconciled. Opium
stimulates the imagination, but cannot *create*

THE MILK OF PARADISE

a strong imaginative faculty where none has existed before. As Parish explains, "The sensory deceptions vary in character with the imaginative power of the individual" (*Hallucinations*, p. 189). Some addicts feel only the "negative pleasure" of physical relief; the "positive pleasure" of vision is reserved for the fortunate few already rich in imaginative equipment. (See Lawrence Kolb, "Pleasure and Deterioration from Narcotic Addiction," *Journal of Mental Hygiene*, IX (1926) 699.)

Ludlow tells of two friends one of whom experienced rich visions upon taking hasheesh, although the other felt only the negative effects of physical pleasure (*The Hasheesh Eater*, pp. 102–107).

41. It remained for Arthur Ainger, in 1903, to ascribe to opium any influence upon Crabbe's work. (See *Crabbe*, "English Men of Letters," London, 1903, pp. 84–85, 88–89).
42. Although the son is lax as to dates, Ainger places the event in this year (*Crabbe*, p. 79).
43. *Cf.* note 19, above.
44. George Crabbe, *The Life of the Rev. George Crabbe*, Cambridge, 1834, pp. 153–154. The analysis was over-optimistic.
45. Extract from a Journal of July 21, 1817 (Crabbe, *Life*, p. 243). That Crabbe admitted using scenes from his dreams in his poetry appears in a letter from J. G. Lockhart to the younger Crabbe (*Life*, p. 270).
46. Ainger, *Crabbe*, p. 177.
47. *Ibid.*, pp. 79–80.
48. *Poetical Works of the Rev. George Crabbe*, ed. by his son (George Crabbe), London, 1834,

NOTES

IV, 116 ff. The poem was found undated in a manuscript (Ainger, *Crabbe*, p. 88).

49. "I was hardly sensible of my feet touching the ground; it seemed as if my feet slid along the ground, impelled by some individual agent, and that my blood was composed of some ethereal fluid, which rendered my body lighter than air." (D. W. Cheever, "Narcotics," *North American Review*, XCV [1862], 388.)
50. See DeQuincey, *Writings*, III, 435.
51. Ainger (p. 78) dates it in 1804–1805.
52. *Work of George Crabbe*, II, 261 ff.
53. Havelock Ellis, *The World of Dreams*, London, 1926, p. 33.
54. Charles Baudelaire, *Edgar Poe*, Paris, 1885, p. 31. For similar light phenomena in Crabbe's own dreams, see "World of Dreams," stanza xxx.
55. *Les Opiomanes*, p. 94. Arthur Symons, the author of "The Opium Smoker," in another poem, "The Crisis," exhibiting all the characteristics of opium dream persecution, describes the brilliant pain of light (*Days and Nights*, London, 1889, pp. 99 ff.). Close in detail to Crabbe's descriptions are the "scattered flash of lights, leaping, and whirled, and mixed inextricably"; and the following:

    Suddenly forth
    Sprang from the farthest clouds and leaped and flashed
    Cleaving and shearing through the veil of rain
    Incessant arrows of the lightning.

56. George Saintsbury, *Essays in English Literature*, London, 1890, "Crabbe," p. 21.

57. In "The Hall of Justice" is a stanza which may be reminiscent of his dreams of terror. See *Works*, II, 287.
58. See John Livingston Lowes, *Convention and Revolt in Poetry*, Cambridge, Massachusetts, 1931, p. 131.
59. For Crabbe's verse forms, see Hermann Pesta, *George Crabbe, Eine Würdigung Seiner Werke*, Wien and Leipzig, 1899, pp. 60, 71 ff.
60. *Life*, p. 252.
61. See Terry and Peelens, *The Opium Problem*, pp. 62–63, 100.
62. Everard Meynell, *The Life of Francis Thompson*, New York, 1926, p. 37.
63. For the interesting question of how deeply the desire for drugs may have been innate in these poets, see Dupouy, p. 299; Cocteau, p. 151; and especially, Benno Hahn, *Die Morphin-Erkrankungen*, Heidelberg, 1927, pp. 59–62.
64. Meynell, *Life*, p. 39.
65. *Ibid.*, p. 44.
66. *Ibid.*, p. 45.
67. *Ibid.*, p. 58.
68. *Ibid.*, p. 75.
69. *Ibid.*, p. 273.
70. *Ibid,*, p. 264. Cf. *Confessions*, Garnett edition, p. 263.
71. Jeannette Marks, *Genius and Disaster*, New York, 1925, p. 41.
72. *Works of Francis Thompson*, New York, 1913, I, 8–9. As an example of likenesses to opium imagery, the autobiographical "Sister Songs" is a good example (*Works*, I, 25 ff.). For eternal persecution, see p. 36; for fluidity of

NOTES

outline, p. 31, and cf. Dupouy, p. 94; for light phenomena, pp. 31–32; for sound, p. 28; and for monsters, p. 45.

73. *Works*, III, 118.
74. Arthur Symons furnishes still another close parallel in his "Andante of Snakes" (*The Fool of the World and Other Poems*, London, 1906, p. 81), in the rich colors and flection of light, and even in the figure of snakes to express it. Here are a few lines only:

They weave a slow andante as in sleep.
Scaled yellow, swampy black, plague-spotted white . . .
                      Woven intricacies
Of Oriental arabesques awake,
Unfold, expand, contract, and raise and sway,

then

Droop back to stagnant immobility.

Ludlow too, pp. 34–38, records a somewhat similar hasheesh phenomenon.

    The heavy paneling of the walls was adorned with grotesque frescoes of every imaginable bird, beast, and monster, which, by some hidden law of life and motion, were forever changing, like the figures of the kaleidoscope.

Cf. also DeQuincey's vision, p. 10, above.
75. Dupouy, p. 93.
76. *Works*, III, 120–121.
77. Crabbe had this experience, when he saw the "female fiend" in the "World of Dreams" (*Poems*, IV, 118). "Why fixed on me that eye of stone?" he cries. Closer still is Symons's "Crisis." In addition to the sea of twisting

faces that DeQuincy saw, Symons notes the accusing eyes through eternity:

> Faces in the dark,
> Through the hot-throbbing age-long nights ...
>
> Staring upon him with *wide opened* eyes,
> Eyes of an *ageless* agony endured, —
> Faces absorbed upon a sea of mist,
> Still, tossing, floating, shuddering, intertwined
> Going and coming.
>
> (*Days and Nights*, p. 102. Italics mine.)

78. *Works*, III, 125–126.
79. *Ibid.*
80. *Ibid.*
81. *Ibid.*, p. 127.
82. *Ibid.*, p. 135. Again, *cf.* Symons's "Crisis": "the haunting thought," which tracked him and "crept up, as with a *hot breath on his neck.*"
83. See Appendix.
84. See *The Road to Xanadu*, Boston and New York, 1930. The Note Book is a "small manuscript volume of ninety leaves," embracing a period from the spring of 1795 to the summer of 1798. (Lowes, *Xanadu*, p. 5). It is *add. MSS.* 27901, in the British Museum, and has been reprinted in a faulty edition by Aloys Brandl, "S. T. Coleridge's Notizbuch aus den Jahren 1795–1798," *Archiv für das Studium der Neueren Sprachen*, XCVII (1896), pp. 332 ff.
85. *The Road to Xanadu*, p. 191.
86. *Ibid.*
87. Lowes's reading, *Xanadu*, p. 517. Brandl reads "pang" (*Archiv*, p. 369).

NOTES

88. *Note Book*, fols. 77b, 77a; *Archiv*, p. 369.
89. They begin fol. 75b, and continue through fol. 78a (*Xanadu*, p. 517).
90. *Poetical Works of Samuel Taylor Coleridge*, ed. James Dykes Campbell, London, 1893, pp. 457-458.
91. *Xanadu*, p. 517.
92. *Archiv*, p. 337.
93. See Appendix.
94. The passage occurs on fol. 27b (*Archiv*, p. 346); the excerpt from the "Ode" on fol. 28b (*Archiv*, p. 356).
95. Fol. 29a; *Archiv*, p. 357.
96. *Ibid*.
97. Fol. 53b; *Archiv*, p. 364. An interesting example of a shot in the dark striking home is Brandl's guess about these jottings, based on the single reference to "an opium chewer"; "*Vermutlich war auch Opium mit im Spiel*" (*Archiv*, p. 337). I discovered this hypothesis only after my own investigations had led me to a similar opinion.
98. *Archiv*, p. 337. Again Brandl struck near the truth when he called the Note Book the "pathologische Kommentär" to these lines, and attributed them to "seelische Überhitzheit," not "dichterische Übertreibung."
99. *Cf*. DeQuincey's *Writings*, III, 447.
100. *Complete Poetical Works of Samuel Taylor Coleridge*, ed. Ernest Hartley Coleridge, Oxford, 1912, p. 389.
101. Preface to "Kubla Khan," *ibid*., p. 297.
102. *Memorials of Coleorton*, ed. William Knight, Boston and New York, 1887, p. 7.
103. Before leaving the subject of Coleridge's

dreams of horror, I must mention a few lines in "The Visionary Hope" (?1810) which seem to describe the same experiences of "obscure pangs," and "dreaded sleep . . . each night scattered by its own loud screams" (*Poetical Works*, p. 416).

104. *Xanadu*, p. 139.
105. *New Essays towards a Critical Method*, London, 1897, p. 187.
106. *Ibid.*, p. 138.
107. See *Xanadu*, pp. 414 ff.
108. *Letters of Samuel Taylor Coleridge*, ed. Ernest Hartley Coleridge, London, 1895, I, 222-223.
109. *Xanadu*, p. 420.
110. *Ibid.*, p. 422.
111. *Ibid.*, p. 425.
112. Prefatory note to "We Are Seven," in *Memories of William Wordsworth*, ed. Christopher Wordsworth, London, 1851, I, 107-108.
113. Campbell, *Poems*, p. 594.
114. DeQuincey's *Writings*, II, 145. It is important that DeQuincey is attacking Coleridge for denying Shelvocke's albatross as a source for "The Ancient Mariner"; and thus this statement weakens his own case!
115. *Xanadu*, p. 136.
116. George Crabbe, *Poetical Works*, "The Village," II, 76.
117. It is interesting that both "Sir Eustace" and "The Ancient Mariner" utilize polar scenery. Sir Eustace felt the "icy wound" through "all that half-year's polar night"; and, in Coleridge's poem, the "wondrous cold" and "ice, mast high" play an impor-

tant part. Walter Cotton, *Knickerbocker*, VII (1836), 422, describes a vision in which he had been frozen upon an iceberg. Some light may be thrown on the causes of these phenomena by DeQuincey's descriptions of the feeling of great cold caused by an undersupply of opium (*Writings*, XIV, 275–276).

118. Another bit of evidence which may be significant appears in the sub-title, "A Poet's Reverie," appended to the 1800 edition of the poem (*Xanadu*, p. 306). Mr. Lowes's explanation is that this was added to ward off the accusation of improbability from Mrs. Barbauld and her kind. Might it not refer rather to the opium revery in which the material for the poem first took shape?

119. *Confessions, Athenaeum Edition*, pp. 239–240.

120. Mr. Lowes mentions this possibility. See *Xanadu*, pp. 418, 425.

121. *Xanadu*, pp. 343 ff.

122. The problem why so unimportant a crime should have such dire consequences has long been a matter of discussion. (For example, see *Xanadu*, pp. 298–303.) Comparison with opium dreams by other authors offers an explanation, at least in part. In many descriptions of opium persecution — and this is true for those which are merely descriptive, as well as those which were later fitted with a crime for motivation — there is, to be sure, a sense of guilt, yet also a feeling that the punishment is *undeserved*. In the "World of Dreams," although "it is his sin" which begins the torment, Crabbe "per-

THE MILK OF PARADISE

ceives and yet endures *the wrong*." In "Sir Eustace" occurs: "Harmless I was, yet hunted down, for treasons to my soul unfit." The persecutions of Symons's "The Crisis," although attending "a deadly sin," are later said to follow "the shadow of a *fancied* crime." In Coleridge's own "Pains of Sleep" he cries that "all seemed guilt, remorse or woe"; yet, he asks, though these punishments may befit others, "wherefore, wherefore fall on me?"

123. The colors are close to those described in the opium passage of the Note Book. It is interesting that Mr. Lowes, without knowing the source of these appearances, suggested that the colors "may have been at least a contributory blue in the nebulous mass which finally took form in the auroral lightings of the Mariner's sky" (*Xanadu*, pp. 191-192).

124. The following is a part of the long passage on the "sweet sounds" which rise as the seraphs leave the corpses:

> Around, around, flew each sweet sound.
> Then darted to the Sun;
> Slowly the sounds came back again,
> Now mixed, now one by one. . . .
>
> Sometimes all little birds that are,
> How they seemed to fill the sea and air
> With their sweet jargoning!
>
> And now 'twas like all instruments,
> Now like a lonely flute.

If there is doubt whether the uncertain flection, the abnormal sweetness, and the intense acuteness of these sounds originated in a narcotic state of hearing, I add bits from

NOTES

a similar passage in Thompson's "Sister Songs":

> I heard a dainty dubious sound
>   As of goodly melody;
> Which first was faint as if in swound,
>   Then burst so suddenly
> In warring concord all around
> That whence this thing might be,
>   To see
> The very marrow longed in me! . . .
>
> So heavenly flutes made murmerous plain
> To heavenly viols, that again
>   — Aching with music — wailed back pain;
> Regals release their notes, which rise
>   Welling, like tears from heart to eyes.

125. Quoted in *Complete Poetical Works of Samuel Taylor Coleridge*, ed. E. H. Coleridge, Oxford, 1912, I, 204, note. (From the *Lyrical Ballads* edition of the poem, 1798.)
126. Comparisons may be made between:
    1. Thirst, and Ludlow, pp. 59 and 72;
    2. "Death" and "Life in Death," and Crabbe's spectres ("World of Dreams," stanza III);
    3. The sensation of lightness and floating, and Ludlow, pp. 26–27, and Crabbe's "World of Dreams."
127. *Xanadu*, p. 407.
128. For the usual version see "Apologia pro Vita Sua," *Poetical Works*, ed. E. H. Coleridge, I, 345.
129. See *Xanadu*, p. 407.
130. "Genial hour" was substituted for "tipsy hour" in the later version. Coleridge cer-

tainly was referring to opium, not alcohol. Wine is not conducive to exaltation of space.

131. Coleridge wrote "the summer of 1787"; but 1798, according to E. H. Coleridge, *Poetical Works*, I, 295, note, is the correct date.
132. This is proved by Coleridge's own manuscript note. See *Xanadu*, p. 417; *Letters*, ed. E. H. Coleridge, I, 245, note; *Poetical Works*, I, 295, note.
133. Coleridge's preface to "Kubla Khan," *Poetical Works*, I, 295–296.
134. Havelock Ellis in the *World of Dreams* (p. 275), doubts whether in a real dream Coleridge could have recalled more than one or two lines. In my opinion, "sleep" is as ambiguous as "anodyne." Coleridge should have written "opium revery," which is a different thing from an actual dream. This would explain away the difficulty, for composition in an "opium revery" could still be conscious enough to be remembered, yet have all the flux and other characteristics of the opium vision (Dupouy, 99 ff.) Cocteau tells of a dramatic scenario composed in such a state, and later recollected in detail, dialogue and all (*Opium*, p. 149).
135. See *Xanadu*, pp. 406–409, for an understanding of how tremendous were the shifts to widely disparate images from Coleridge's reading.
136. *Ibid.*, pp. 407–408.
137. Mrs. Barbauld's statement, quoted in *Xanadu*, pp. 301–302.
138. The judgment expressed by Jeanette Marks, *Genius and Disaster*, New York, 1925, pp.

NOTES

169–170, is typical. She puts the issue thus: "Is drug mentality to set a standard for English poetry and prose? Is drug imagination to be the matrix on which we shape the imaginative powers?" If not, "it means a revision of our list of so-called 'classics' by the help of the literary alienist or pathologist. The other way it means a clear-eyed acceptance of the abnormal, of the diseased, of the morbid, as pacemaker in what we call our best literary achievements."

139. See John Livingston Lowes, *Convention and Revolt in Poetry*, Boston and New York, 1919, pp. 98 ff.
140. See George Saintsbury, *A History of Nineteenth Century Literature*, London, 1927, p. 62.
141. *Writings*, III, 206.
142. See *ibid.*, III, 433; and the Garnett edition, p. 264.
143. See *Confessions, Athenaeum Press*, pp. 233–234, and Campbell, *Coleridge*, pp. 128, 137.
144. After the great period of the "Mariner," "Kubla Khan," and "Christabel, Part I," Coleridge wrote little which again attained so high a standard. The evidence of opium in "Christabel" or any later work is not prominent enough to warrant further treatment.
145. See *Unpublished Letters*, II, 111.

Notes to Appendix

1. *Unpublished Letters*, I, 3.
2. *Xanadu*, p. 415.
3. See note 19, above.

4. E. H. C., *Letters*, I, 14–15.
5. Campbell, *Life*, p. 14.
6. *Poems*, I, 17.
7. Campbell, *Life*, p. 23.
8. *Letters*, ed. E. H. Coleridge, I, 45.
9. *Unpublished Letters*, I, 7.
10. *Ibid.*, I, 28.
11. *Ibid.*, I, 45.
12. *Letters*, ed. E. H. Coleridge, I, 154–155.
13. *Ibid.*, I, 156.
14. Hahn, *Die Morphin-Erkrangungen*, pp. 59 ff.
15. See below, p. 59.
16. *Xanadu*, p. 417.
17. *Letters*, ed. E. H. Coleridge, pp. 173–175.
18. *Xanadu*, p. 604h, 604i.
19. *Ibid.*
20. Quoted in *Xanadu*, p. 518.
21. *Letters*, ed. E. H. Coleridge, I, 193.
22. *Ibid.*, I, 209.
23. *Xanadu*, p. 518.
24. *Unpublished Letters*, I, 70.
25. *Letters*, ed. E. H. Coleridge, pp. 228–229.
26. *Letters*, ed. E. H. Coleridge, p. 240.
27. For evidence from sources outside Coleridge's letters that his recourse to opium was even more habitual than his letters indicate, see *Xanadu*, pp. 599–600.

BIBLIOGRAPHY

BIBLIOGRAPHY

DISCUSSIONS OF OPIUM PHENOMENA

Cheever, D. W., "Narcotics," *North American Review*, XCV (1862), 374–415.

Cotton, Walter, "Turkish Sketches — Effects of Opium," *The Knickerbocker*, vii (1836), 421–423.

Dupouy, Roger, *Les Opiomanes*, Paris, 1912.

Hahn, Benno, *Die Morphin-Erkrangungen*, Heidelberg, 1927.

Lewin, Louis, *Phantastica*, London, 1931.

Marks, Jeannette, *Genius and Disaster*, New York, 1925.

The Opium Habit, Anonymous, New York, 1868.

Terry, Charles E., and Peelens, Mildred, *The Opium Problem*, New York, 1928.

SAMUEL TAYLOR COLERIDGE

Coleridge, *Complete Poetical Works*, ed. Ernest Hartley Coleridge, Oxford, 1912.

Coleridge, *Letters*, ed. Ernest Hartley Coleridge, London, 1895.

Coleridge, *Unpublished Letters*, ed. Earl Leslie Griggs, London, 1932.

Coleridge, *Memorials of Coleorton*, ed. William Knight, Cambridge, 1887.

Brandl, Aloys, "S. T. Coleridge's Notizbuch aus den Jahren 1795–1798," *Archiv für das Studium der Neueren Sprachen*, XCVII (1896), 332 ff.

Campbell, James Dykes, *Samuel Taylor Coleridge*, London, 1894.

Lowes, John Livingston, *The Road to Xanadu*, Cambridge, 1930.

Memoirs of William Wordsworth, ed. Christopher Wordsworth, London, 1851.

Robertson, John Mackinnon, *New Essays towards a Critical Method*, London, 1897.

GEORGE CRABBE

Crabbe, *Poetical Works*, ed. George Crabbe, London, 1834.

Ainger, Alfred, *Crabbe* (English Men of Letters), London, 1903.

Crabbe, George, *Life of the Rev. George Crabbe*, Cambridge and Boston, 1834.

Kebble, T. E., *Life of George Crabbe*, London, 1888.

Pesta, Hermann, *George Crabbe*, Vienna and Leipzig, 1899.

Saintsbury, George, "Crabbe," *Essays in English Literature*, London, 1890.

THOMAS DEQUINCEY

DeQuincey, *Collected Writings*, London, 1896.

DeQuincey, *Confessions of An English Opium-Eater*, ed. Richard Garnett, London, 1895.

DeQuincey, *Selections*, ed. M. H. Turk (Athenaeum Press Series), Boston, 1902.

Masson, David, *DeQuincey*, London, 1926.

EDGAR ALLAN POE

Poe, *Works*, ed. Edmund Clarence Stedman and George Edward Woodberry, New York, 1906.

Allen, Hervey, *Israfel*, New York, 1926.

BIBLIOGRAPHY

Ingram, John H., *Edgar Allan Poe*, London, 1880.
Menz, Lotte, *Die sinnlichen Elemente bei Edgar Allan Poe*, Doctoral Dissertation, Marburg, 1915.
Pollak, Simon, *Edgar Poe — un Génie Toxicomane*, Paris, 1928.
Robertson, John S., *Edgar A. Poe*, New York, 1923.
Weiss, Susan Archer, *Home Life of Poe*, New York, 1907.
Woodberry, George E., *Life of Edgar Allan Poe*, Cambridge, 1909.

Francis Thompson

Thompson, *Works*, New York, 1913.
Meynell, Edward, *Life of Francis Thompson*, New York, 1926.

James Thomson

Thomson, *Life and Poetry*, ed. J. Edward Meeker, New Haven, 1907.
Salt, H. S., *Life of James Thomson* ("B. V."), London, 1914.
Worcester, David, *James Thomson the Second*, Doctoral Dissertation (unprinted), Harvard University, 1933.

Miscellaneous

Bates, William Nickerson, Jr., *Poetical Intoxication*, Cambridge, 1930.
Baudelaire, Charles, *Ouevres Complètes*, ed. Jacques Crepet, Paris, 1922.
Baudelaire, *Petits Poèmes en Prose*, Paris, 1869.
Baudelaire, *Edgar Poe*, Paris, 1885.
Cocteau, Jean, *Opium*, New York, 1932.

THE MILK OF PARADISE

Cutten, George B., *Psychology of Alcoholism*, New York, 1907.

Ellis, Havelock, *The World of Dreams*, London, 1926.

Lowes, John Livingston, *Convention and Revolt in Poetry*, Boston and New York, 1931.

Ludlow, Fitzhugh, *The Hasheesh Eater*, New York, 1857.

Parish, Edmund, *Hallucinations and Illusions*, London, 1897.

Saintsbury, George, *History of Nineteenth Century Literature*, London, 1927.

Symons, Azthur, *Days and Nights*, London and New York, 1889.

Symons, *The Fool of the World and Other Poems*, London, 1906.

APPENDIX TO THE PERENNIAL LIBRARY EDITION

For the benefit of the reader, the text has been supplemented with the rarer items among those discussed in the book. Coleridge's poems are widely known—and widely available in various paperback editions—and De Quincey's *Confessions of an English Opium Eater* is a book in itself and accessible in two paperback editions, Signet and Everyman.

Reprinted below are two poems by George Crabbe, "The World of Dreams" and "Sir Eustace Grey" (taken from *The Poetical Works*, edited by A. J. and R. M. Carlyle, 1914) and a prose piece by Francis Thompson, "Finis Coronat Opus" (taken from *The Works of Francis Thompson*, edited by Wilfrid Meynell, 3 volumes, 1913).

George Crabbe

The World of Dreams

THE WORLD OF DREAMS

[Date uncertain]

I

And is thy soul so wrapt in sleep?
  Thy senses, thy affections, fled?
No play of fancy thine, to keep
  Oblivion from that grave, thy bed?
Then art thou but the breathing dead:
  I envy, but I pity too:
The bravest may *my* terrors dread,
  The happiest fain *my* joys pursue.

II

Soon as the real World I lose,
  Quick Fancy takes her wonted way,
Or Baxter's sprites my soul abuse—
  For how it is I cannot say,
Nor to what powers a passive prey,
  I feel such bliss, I fear such pain;
But all is gloom, or all is gay,
  Soon as th' ideal World I gain.

III

Come, then, I woo thee, sacred Sleep!
  Vain troubles of the world, farewell!
Spirits of Ill! your distance keep—
  And in your own dominions dwell,

Ye, the sad emigrants from hell !
  Watch, dear seraphic beings, round,
And these black Enemies repel ;
  Safe be my soul, my slumbers sound !

IV

In vain I pray ! It is my sin
  That thus admits the shadowy throng.
Oh ! now they break tumultuous in—
  Angels of darkness fierce and strong.
Oh ! I am borne of fate along ;
  My soul, subdued, admits the foe,
Perceives and yet endures the wrong,
  Resists, and yet prepares to go.

V

Where am I now ? and what to meet ?
  Where I have been entrapt before :
The wicked city's vilest street,—
  I know what I must now explore.
The dark-brow'd throng more near and more,
  With murderous looks are on me thrust,
And lo ! they ope the accursed door,
  And I must go—I know I must !

VI

That female fiend !—Why is she there ?
  Alas ! I know her.—Oh, begone !
Why is that tainted bosom bare,
  Why fix'd on me that eye of stone ?
Why have they left us thus alone ?
  I saw the deed—why then appear ?
Thou art not form'd of blood and bone !
  Come not, dread being, come not near !

VII

So ! all is quiet, calm, serene ;
  I walk a noble mansion round—
From room to room, from scene to scene,
  I breathless pass, in gloom profound :
No human shape, no mortal sound—
  I feel an awe, I own a dread,
And still proceed !—nor stop nor bound—
  And all is silent, all is dead.

VIII

Now I'm hurried, borne along,
   All is business! all alive!
Heavens! how mighty is the throng,
   Voices humming like a hive!
Through the swelling crowd I strive,
   Bustling forth my way to trace:
Never fated to arrive
   At the still-expected place.

IX

Ah me! how sweet the morning sun
   Deigns on yon sleepy town to shine!
How soft those far-off rivers run—
   Those trees their leafy heads decline!
Balm-breathing zephyrs, all divine,
   Their health-imparting influence give:
Now, all that earth allows is mine—
   Now, now I dream not, but I live.

X

My friend my brother, lost in youth,
   I meet in doubtful, glad surprise,
In conscious love, in fearless truth:
   What pleasures in the meeting rise!
Ah! brief enjoyment!—Pleasure dies
   E'en in its birth, and turns to pain:
He meets me with hard glazèd eyes!
   He quits me—spurns me—with disdain.

XI

I sail the sea, I walk the land;
   In all the world am I alone:
Silent I pace the sea-worn sand,
   Silent I view the princely throne;
I listen heartless for the tone
   Of winds and waters, but in vain;
Creation dies without a groan!
   And I without a hope remain!

XII

Unnumber'd riches I behold,
 Glories untasted I survey:
My heart is sick, my bosom cold,
 Friends! neighbours! kindred! where are they?
In the sad, last, long, endless day!
 When I can neither pray nor weep,
Doom'd o'er the sleeping world to stray,
 And not to die, and not to sleep.

XIII

Beside the summer sea I stand,
 Where the slow billows swelling shine:
How beautiful this pearly sand,
 That waves, and winds, and years refine:
Be this delicious quiet mine!
 The joy of youth! so sweet before,
When I could thus my frame recline,
 And watch th' entangled weeds ashore.

XIV

Yet, I remember not that sea,
 That other shore on yonder side:
Between them narrow bound must be,
 If equal rise th' opposing tide—
Lo! lo! they rise—and I abide
 The peril of the meeting flood:
Away, away, my footsteps slide—
 I pant upon the clinging mud!

XV

Oh let me now possession take
 Of this—it cannot be a dream.
Yes! now the soul must be awake—
 These pleasures are—they do not seem.
And is it true? Oh joy extreme!
 All whom I loved, and thought them dead,
Far down in Lethe's flowing stream,
 And, with them, life's best pleasures fled:

XVI

Yes, many a tear for them I shed—
   Tears that relieve the anxious breast;
And now, by heavenly favour led,
   We meet—and One, the fairest, best,
Among them—ever-welcome guest!
   Within the room, that seem'd destroy'd—
This room endear'd, and still possess'd,
   By this dear party still enjoy'd.

XVII

Speak to me! speak! that I may know
   I am thus happy!—dearest, speak!
Those smiles that haunt fond memory show!
   Joy makes us doubtful, wavering, weak;
But yet 'tis joy—And all I seek
   Is mine! What glorious day is this!
Now let me bear with spirit meek
   An hour of pure and perfect bliss.

XVIII

But do ye look indeed as friends?
   Is there no change? Are not ye cold?
Oh! I do dread that Fortune lends
   Fictitious good!—that I behold,
To lose, these treasures, which of old
   Were all my glory, all my pride:
May not these arms that form infold?
   Is all affection asks denied?

XIX

Say, what is this?—How are we tried,
   In this sad world!—I know not these—
All strangers, none to me allied—
   Those aspects blood and spirit freeze:
Dear forms, my wandering judgment spare;
   And thou, most dear, these fiends disarm,
Resume thy wonted looks and air,
   And break this melancholy charm.

XX

And are they vanish'd ? Is she lost ?
  Shall never day that form restore ?
Oh ! I am all by fears engross'd ;
  Sad truth has broken in once more,
And I the brief delight deplore :
  How durst they such resemblance take ?
Heavens ! with what grace the mask they wore !
  Oh, from what visions I awake !

XXI

Once more, once more upon the shore !
  Now back the rolling ocean flows :
The rocky bed now far before
  On the receding water grows—
The treasures and the wealth it owes
  To human misery—all in view ;
Fate all on me at once bestows,
  From thousands robb'd and murder'd too.

XXII

But, lo ! whatever I can find
  Grows mean and worthless as I view :
They promise, but they cheat the mind,
  As promises are born to do.
How lovely every form and hue,
  Till seized and master'd—Then arise,
For all that admiration drew,
  All that our senses can despise !

XXIII

Within the basis of a tower,
  I saw a plant—it graced the spot ;
There was within nor wind nor shower,
  And this had life that flowers have not.
I drew it forth—Ah, luckless lot !
  It was the mandrake ; and the sound
Of anguish deeply smother'd shot
  Into my breast with pang profound.

XXIV

' I would I were a soaring bird,'
  Said Folly, ' and I then would fly:
Some mocking Muse or Fairy heard—
  ' You can but fall—suppose you try?
And though you may not mount the sky,
  You will not grovel in the mire.'
Hail, words of comfort! Now can I
  Spurn earth, and to the air aspire.

XXV

And this, before, might I have done
  If I had courage—that is all:
'Tis easier now to soar than run;
  Up! up!—we neither tire nor fall.
Children of dust, be yours to crawl
  On the vile earth!—while, happier, I
Must listen to an inward call,
  That bids me mount, that makes me fly.

XXVI

I tumble from the loftiest tower,
  Yet evil have I never found;
Supported by some favouring power,
  I come in safety to the ground.
I rest upon the sea, the sound
  Of many waters in mine ear,
Yet have no dread of being drown'd,
  But see my way, and cease to fear.

XXVII

Awake, there is no living man
  Who may my fixèd spirit shake;
But, sleeping, there is one who can,
  And oft does he the trial make:
Against his might resolves I take,
  And him oppose with high disdain;
But quickly all my powers forsake
  My mind, and I resume my chain.

XXVIII

I know not how, but I am brought
  Into a large and Gothic hall,
Seated with those I never sought—
  Kings, Caliphs, Kaisers,—silent all;
Pale as the dead; enrobed and tall,
  Majestic, frozen, solemn, still;
They wake my fears, my wits appal,
  And with both scorn and terror fill.

XXIX

Now are they seated at a board
  In that cold grandeur—I am there.
But what can mummied kings afford?
  This is their meagre ghostly fare,
And proves what fleshless things they stare!
  Yes! I am seated with the dead:
How great, and yet how mean they are!
  Yes! I can scorn them while I dread.

XXX

They're gone!—and in their room I see
  A fairy being, form and dress
Brilliant as light; nor can there be
  On earth that heavenly loveliness;
Nor words can that sweet look express,
  Or tell what living gems adorn
That wond'rous beauty: who can guess
  Where such celestial charms were born?

XXXI

Yet, as I wonder and admire,
  The grace is gone, the glory dead;
And now it is but mean attire
  Upon a shrivel'd beldame spread,
Laid loathsome on a pauper's bed,
  Where wretchedness and woe are found,
And the faint putrid odour shed
  By all that's foul and base around!

XXXII

A garden this? oh! lovely breeze!
  Oh! flowers that with such freshness
    bloom!—
Flowers shall I call such forms as these,
  Or this delicious air perfume?
Oh! this from better worlds must come;
  On earth such beauty who can meet?
No! this is not the native home
  Of things so pure, so bright, so sweet!

XXXIII

Where? where?—am I reduced to this—
  Thus sunk in poverty extreme?
Can I not these vile things dismiss?
  No! they are things that more than seem:
This room with that cross-parting beam
  Holds yonder squalid tribe and me—
But they were ever thus, nor dream
  Of being wealthy, favour'd, free!—

XXXIV

Shall I a coat and badge receive,
  And sit among these crippled men,
And not go forth without the leave
  Of him—and ask it humbly then—
Who reigns in this infernal den—
  Where all beside in woe repine?
Yes, yes, I must: nor tongue nor pen
  Can paint such misery as mine!

XXXV

Wretches! if ye were only poor,
  You would my sympathy engage;
Or were ye vicious, and no more,
  I might be fill'd with manly rage;
Or had ye patience, wise and sage
  We might such worthy sufferers call:
But ye are birds that suit your cage—
  Poor, vile, impatient, worthless all!

XXXVI

How came I hither? Oh, that Hag!
  'Tis she the enchanting spell prepares;
By cruel witchcraft she can drag
  My struggling being in her snares:
Oh, how triumphantly she glares!
  But yet would leave me, could I make
Strong effort to subdue my cares.—
  'TIS MADE!—and I to Freedom wake!

George Crabbe

Sir Eustace Grey

SIR EUSTACE GREY

[1807]

SCENE—A MAD-HOUSE

PERSONS—Visitor, Physician, and Patient

> Veris miscens falsa.—
> SENECA, *in Herc. furente*, v. 1070.

VISITOR

I'll know no more;—the heart is torn
By views of wo, we cannot heal;
Long shall I see these things forlorn,
   And oft again their griefs shall feel,
   As each upon the mind shall steal;
That wan projector's mystic style,
   That lumpish idiot leering by,
That peevish idler's ceaseless wile,
And that poor maiden's half-form'd smile,
   While struggling for the full-drawn sigh!
I'll know no more.

PHYSICIAN

               —Yes, turn again;
Then speed to happier scenes thy way,
   When thou hast view'd, what yet remain,
The ruins of Sir Eustace Grey,
   The sport of madness, misery's prey:
But he will no historian need,
   His cares, his crimes, will he display,
And show (as one from frenzy freed)
   The proud-lost mind, the rash-done deed.
That cell to him is Greyling Hall:—
   Approach; he'll bid thee welcome there;
Will sometimes for his servant call,
   And sometimes point the vacant chair:

He can, with free and easy air,
   Appear attentive and polite;
Can veil his woes in manners fair,
   And pity with respect excite.

PATIENT

Who comes?—Approach!—'tis kindly done:—
My learn'd physician, and a friend,
Their pleasures quit, to visit one,
   Who cannot to their ease attend,
Nor joys bestow, nor comforts lend,
   As when I lived so bless'd, so well,
And dreamt not I must soon contend
   With those malignant powers of hell.

PHYSICIAN

Less warmth, Sir Eustace, or we go.—

PATIENT

See! I am calm as infant-love,
A very child, but one of wo,
   Whom you should pity, not reprove:—
But men at ease, who never strove
   With passions wild, will calmly show
How soon we may their ills remove,
   And masters of their madness grow.

Some twenty years I think are gone,—
   (Time flies, I know not how, away,)
The sun upon no happier shone,
   Nor prouder man, than Eustace Grey.
Ask where you would, and all would say,
   The man admired and praised of all,
By rich and poor, by grave and gay,
   Was the young lord of Greyling Hall.

Yes! I had youth and rosy health;
 Was nobly form'd, as man might be;
For sickness then, of all my wealth,
 I never gave a single fee:
The ladies fair, the maidens free,
 Were all accustom'd then to say,
Who would a handsome figure see
 Should look upon Sir Eustace Grey.

He had a frank and pleasant look,
 A cheerful eye and accent bland;
His very speech and manner spoke
 The generous heart, the open hand;
About him all was gay or grand,
 He had the praise of great and small;
He bought, improved, projected, plann'd,
 And reign'd a prince at Greyling Hall.

My lady!—she was all we love;
 All praise (to speak her worth) is faint;
Her manners show'd the yielding dove,
 Her morals, the seraphic saint;
She never breathed nor look'd complaint;
 No equal upon earth had she:—
Now, what is this fair thing I paint?
 Alas! as all that live shall be.

There was, beside, a gallant youth,
 And him my bosom's friend I had:—
Oh! I was rich in very truth,
 It made me proud—it made me mad!—
Yes, I was lost—but there was cause!—
 Where stood my tale?—I cannot find—
But I had all mankind's applause,
 And all the smiles of womankind.

There were two cherub-things beside,
   A gracious girl, a glorious boy;
Yet more to swell my full-blown pride,
   To varnish higher my fading joy,
Pleasures were ours without alloy,
   Nay, Paradise,—till my frail Eve
Our bliss was tempted to destroy;
   Deceived and fated to deceive.

But I deserved; for all that time,
   When I was loved, admired, caress'd,
There was within, each secret crime,
   Unfelt, uncancell'd, unconfess'd:
I never then my God address'd,
   In grateful praise or humble prayer;
And if His Word was not my jest!
   (Dread thought!) it never was my care.

I doubted:—fool I was to doubt!
   If that all-piercing eye could see,—
If He who looks all worlds throughout,
   Would so minute and careful be,
As to perceive and punish me:—
   With man I would be great and high,
But with my God so lost, that He,
   In his large view, should pass me by.

Thus bless'd with children, friend, and wife,
   Bless'd far beyond the vulgar lot;
Of all that gladdens human life,
   Where was the good, that I had not?
But my vile heart had sinful spot,
   And Heaven beheld its deep'ning stain;
Eternal justice I forgot,
   And mercy sought not to obtain.

Come near,—I'll softly speak the rest!—
   Alas! 'tis known to all the crowd,
Her guilty love was all confess'd;
   And his, who so much truth avow'd,
My faithless friend's.—In pleasure proud
   I sat, when these cursed tidings came;
Their guilt, their flight was told aloud,
   And Envy smiled to hear my shame!

I call'd on Vengeance; at the word
   She came:—Can I the deed forget?
I held the sword, th' accursed sword,
   The blood of his false heart made wet;
And that fair victim paid her debt,
   She pined, she died, she loath'd to live;—
I saw her dying—see her yet:
   Fair fallen thing! my rage forgive!

Those cherubs still, my life to bless,
   Were left; could I my fears remove,
Sad fears that check'd each fond caress,
   And poison'd all parental love?
Yet that with jealous feelings strove,
   And would at last have won my will,
Had I not, wretch! been doom'd to prove
   Th' extremes of mortal good and ill.

In youth! health! joy! in beauty's pride!
   They droop'd: as flowers when blighted bow,
The dire infection came:—They died,
   And I was cursed—as I am now——
Nay, frown not, angry friend,—allow
   That I was deeply, sorely tried;
Hear then, and you must wonder how
   I could such storms and strifes abide.

Storms!—not that clouds embattled make,
  When they afflict this earthly globe;
But such as with their terrors shake
  Man's breast, and to the bottom probe;
They make the hypocrite disrobe,
  They try us all, if false or true;
For this, one devil had pow'r on Job;
  And I was long the slave of two.

PHYSICIAN

Peace, peace, my friend; these subjects fly;
  Collect thy thoughts—go calmly on.—

PATIENT

And shall I then the fact deny?
  I was,—thou know'st,—I was begone,
Like him who fill'd the eastern throne,
  To whom the Watcher cried aloud [1];
That royal wretch of Babylon,
  Who was so guilty and so proud.

Like him, with haughty, stubborn mind,
  I, in my state, my comforts sought;
Delight and praise I hoped to find,
  In what I builded, planted, bought!
Oh! arrogance! by misery taught—
  Soon came a voice! I felt it come;
'Full be his cup, with evil fraught,
  Demons his guides, and death his doom!'

Then was I cast from out my state;
  Two fiends of darkness led my way;
They waked me early, watch'd me late,
  My dread by night, my plague by day!
Oh! I was made their sport, their play,
  Through many a stormy troubled year;
And how they used their passive prey
  Is sad to tell:—but you shall hear.

And first, before they sent me forth,
　　Through this unpitying world to run,
They robb'd Sir Eustace of his worth,
　　Lands, manors, lordships, every one;
So was that gracious man undone,
　　Was spurn'd as vile, was scorn'd as poor,
Whom every former friend would shun,
　　And menials drove from every door.

Then those ill-favour'd Ones[2], whom none
　　But my unhappy eyes could view,
Led me, with wild emotion, on,
　　And, with resistless terror, drew.
Through lands we fled, o'er seas we flew,
　　And halted on a boundless plain;
Where nothing fed, nor breathed, nor grew,
　　But silence ruled the still domain.

Upon that boundless plain, below,
　　The setting sun's last rays were shed,
And gave a mild and sober glow,
　　Where all were still, asleep, or dead;
Vast ruins in the midst were spread,
　　Pillars and pediments sublime,
Where the grey moss had form'd a bed,
　　And clothed the crumbling spoils of time.

There was I fix'd, I know not how,
　　Condemn'd for untold years to stay:
Yet years were not;—one dreadful *now*
　　Endured no change of night or day;
The same mild evening's sleeping ray
　　Shone softly-solemn and serene,
And all that time I gazed away,
　　The setting sun's sad rays were seen.

At length a moment's sleep stole on,—
　Again came my commission'd foes;
Again through sea and land we're gone,
　No peace, no respite, no repose:
Above the dark broad sea we rose,
　We ran through bleak and frozen land;
I had no strength their strength t' oppose,
　An infant in a giant's hand.

They placed me where those streamers play,
　Those nimble beams of brilliant light;
It would the stoutest heart dismay,
　To see, to feel, that dreadful sight:
So swift, so pure, so cold, so bright,
　They pierced my frame with icy wound,
And all that half-year's polar night,
　Those dancing streamers wrapp'd me round.

Slowly that darkness pass'd away,
　When down upon the earth I fell,—
Some hurried sleep was mine by day;
　But, soon as toll'd the evening bell,
They forced me on, where ever dwell
　Far-distant men in cities fair,
Cities of whom no trav'lers tell,
　Nor feet but mine were wanderers there.

Their watchmen stare, and stand aghast,
　As on we hurry through the dark;
The watch-light blinks as we go past,
　The watch-dog shrinks and fears to bark;
The watch-tower's bell sounds shrill; and, hark!
The free wind blows—we've left the town—
A wide sepulchral-ground I mark,
　And on a tombstone place me down.

What monuments of mighty dead!
　What tombs of various kinds are found!
And stones erect their shadows shed
　On humble graves, with wickers bound;
Some risen fresh, above the ground,
　Some level with the native clay,
What sleeping millions wait the sound,
　' Arise, ye dead, and come away!'

Alas! they stay not for that call;
　Spare me this wo! ye demons, spare!—
They come! the shrouded shadows all,—
　'Tis more than mortal brain can bear;
Rustling they rise, they sternly glare
　At man upheld by vital breath;
Who, led by wicked fiends, should dare
　To join the shadowy troops of death!

Yes, I have felt all man can feel,
　Till he shall pay his nature's debt;
Ills that no hope has strength to heal,
　No mind the comfort to forget:
Whatever cares the heart can fret,
　The spirits wear, the temper gall,
Wo, want, dread, anguish, all beset
　My sinful soul!—together all!

Those fiends upon a shaking fen
　Fix'd me, in dark tempestuous night;
There never trod the foot of men,
　There flock'd the fowl in wint'ry flight;
There danced the moor's deceitful light
　Above the pool where sedges grow;
And when the morning-sun shone bright,
　It shone upon a field of snow.

They hung me on a bough so small,
   The rook could build her nest no higher;
They fix'd me on the trembling ball
   That crowns the steeple's quiv'ring spire;
They set me where the seas retire,
   But drown with their returning tide;
And made me flee the mountain's fire,
   When rolling from its burning side.

I've hung upon the ridgy steep
   Of cliffs, and held the rambling brier;
I've plunged below the billowy deep,
   Where air was sent me to respire;
I've been where hungry wolves retire;
   And (to complete my woes) I've ran
Where Bedlam's crazy crew conspire
   Against the life of reasoning man.

I've furl'd in storms the flapping sail,
   By hanging from the topmast-head;
I've served the vilest slaves in jail,
   And pick'd the dunghill's spoil for bread;
I've made the badger's hole my bed,
   I've wander'd with a gipsy crew;
I've dreaded all the guilty dread,
   And done what they would fear to do.

On sand, where ebbs and flows the flood,
   Midway they placed and bade me die;
Propp'd on my staff, I stoutly stood
   When the swift waves came rolling by;
And high they rose, and still more high,
   Till my lips drank the bitter brine;
I sobb'd convulsed, then cast mine eye,
   And saw the tide's re-flowing sign.

And then, my dreams were such as nought
　　Could yield but my unhappy case;
I've been of thousand devils caught,
　　And thrust into that horrid place,
Where reign dismay, despair, disgrace;
　　Furies with iron fangs were there,
To torture that accursed race,
　　Doom'd to dismay, disgrace, despair.

Harmless I was; yet hunted down
　　For treasons, to my soul unfit;
I've been pursued through many a town,
　　For crimes that petty knaves commit;
I've been adjudged t' have lost my wit,
　　Because I preach'd so loud and well;
And thrown into the dungeon's pit,
　　For trampling on the pit of hell.

Such were the evils, man of sin,
　　That I was fated to sustain;
And add to all, without—within,
　　A soul defiled with every stain
That man's reflecting mind can pain;
　　That pride, wrong, rage, despair, can make
In fact, they'd nearly touch'd my brain,
　　And reason on her throne would shake.

But pity will the vilest seek,
　　If punish'd guilt will not repine,—
I heard a heavenly teacher speak,
　　And felt the SUN OF MERCY shine:
I hail'd the light! the birth divine!
　　And then was seal'd among the few;
Those angry fiends beheld the sign,
　　And from me in an instant flew.

Come hear how thus the charmers cry
  To wandering sheep, the strays of sin,
While some the wicket-gate pass by,
  And some will knock and enter in :
Full joyful 'tis a soul to win,
  For he that winneth souls is wise ;
Now hark ! the holy strains begin,
  And thus the sainted preacher cries :—[3]

' Pilgrim, burthen'd with thy sin,
Come the way to Zion's gate,
There, till Mercy let thee in,
Knock and weep and watch and wait.
  Knock !—He knows the sinner's cry :
  Weep !—He loves the mourner's tears :
  Watch !—for saving grace is nigh :
  Wait,—till heavenly light appears.

' Hark ! it is the Bridegroom's voice ;
Welcome, pilgrim, to thy rest ;
Now within the gate rejoice,
Safe and seal'd and bought and bless'd !
  Safe—from all the lures of vice,
  Seal'd—by signs the chosen know,
  Bought—by love and life the price,
  Bless'd—the mighty debt to owe.

' Holy Pilgrim ! what for thee
In a world like this remain ?
From thy guarded breast shall flee
Fear and shame, and doubt and pain.
  Fear—the hope of Heaven shall fly,
  Shame—from glory's view retire,
  Doubt—in certain rapture die,
  Pain—in endless bliss expire.'

But though my day of grace was come,
 Yet still my days of grief I find ;
The former clouds' collected gloom
 Still sadden the reflecting mind ;
The soul, to evil things consign'd,
 Will of their evil some retain ;
The man will seem to earth inclined,
 And will not look erect again.

Thus, though elect, I feel it hard
 To lose what I possess'd before,
To be from all my wealth debarr'd,—
 The brave Sir Eustace is no more :
But old I wax and passing poor,
 Stern, rugged men my conduct view ;
They chide my wish, they bar my door,
 'Tis hard—I weep—you see I do.—

Must you, my friends, no longer stay ?
 Thus quickly all my pleasures end ;
But I'll remember, when I pray,
 My kind physician and his friend ;
And those sad hours, you deign to spend
 With me, I shall requite them all ;
Sir Eustace for his friends shall send,
 And thank their love at Greyling Hall.

VISITOR

The poor Sir Eustace !—Yet his hope
 Leads him to think of joys again ;
And when his earthly visions droop,
 His views of heavenly kind remain :—
But whence that meek and humbled strain,
 That spirit wounded, lost, resign'd ?
Would not so proud a soul disdain
 The madness of the poorest mind ?

PHYSICIAN

No! for the more he swell'd with pride,
　The more he felt misfortune's blow;
Disgrace and grief he could not hide,
　And poverty had laid him low:
Thus shame and sorrow working slow,
　At length this humble spirit gave;
Madness on these began to grow,
　And bound him to his fiends a slave.

Though the wild thoughts had touch'd his brain,
　Then was he free:—So, forth he ran;
To soothe or threat, alike were vain:
　He spake of fiends; look'd wild and wan;
Year after year, the hurried man
　Obey'd those fiends from place to place;
Till his religious change began
　To form a frenzied child of grace.

For, as the fury lost its strength,
　The mind reposed; by slow degrees
Came lingering hope, and brought at length
　To the tormented spirit, ease:
This slave of sin, whom fiends could seize,
　Felt or believed their power had end;—
' 'Tis faith,' he cried, ' my bosom frees,
　And now my SAVIOUR is my friend.'

But ah! though time can yield relief,
　And soften woes it cannot cure;
Would we not suffer pain and grief,
　To have our reason sound and sure?
Then let us keep our bosoms pure,
　Our fancy's favourite flights suppress;
Prepare the body to endure,
　And bend the mind to meet distress;
And then HIS guardian care implore,
Whom demons dread and men adore.

[112]

Francis Thompson

Finis Coronat Opus

FINIS CORONAT OPUS

IN a city of the future, among a people bearing a name I know not, lived Florentian the poet, whose place was high in the retinue of Fortune. Young, noble, popular, influential, he had succeeded to a rich inheritance, and possessed the natural gifts which gain the love of women. But the seductions which Florentian followed were darker and more baleful than the seductions of women; for they were the seductions of knowledge and intellectual pride. In very early years he had passed from the pursuit of natural to the pursuit of unlawful science; he had conquered power where conquest is disaster, and power servitude.

But the ambition thus gratified had elsewhere suffered check. It was the custom of this people that among their poets he who by universal acclaim outsoared all competitors should be crowned with laurel in public ceremony. Now between Florentian and this distinction there stood a rival. Seraphin was a spirit of higher reach than Florentian, and the time was nearing fast when even the slow eyes of the people must be opened to a supremacy which Florentian himself acknowledged in his own heart. Hence arose in his lawless soul an insane passion; so that all which he had seemed to him as nothing beside that which he had not, and the compassing of this barred achievement became to him the one worthy object of existence. Repeated essay only proved to him the inadequacy of his native genius, and he turned for aid to the power which he served. Nor was the power of evil slow to respond. It promised him assistance that should procure him his heart's desire, but demanded in return a crime before which even the unscrupulous selfishness of Florentian paled. For he had sought and won the hand of Aster, daughter to the Lady Urania, and the sacrifice demanded from him was no other than the sacrifice of his betrothed, the playmate of his childhood. The horror of such a suggestion prevailed for a time over his unslacked ambition. But he, who believed himself a strong worker of ill, was in reality a weak follower of it; he believed himself a Vathek, he was but a Faust: continuous pressure and gradual familiarization could warp him to any sin. Moreover his love for Aster had been gradually and unconsciously sapped by the habitual practice of evil. So God smote Florentian, that his antidote became to him his poison, and love the regenerator love the destroyer. A strong man, he might have been saved by love: a weak man, he was damned by it.

The palace of Florentian was isolated in the environs of the city; and on the night before his marriage he stood in the room known to his domestics as the Chamber of Statues. Both its appearance, and the sounds which (his servants averred) sometimes issued from it, contributed to secure for him the seclusion that he desired whenever he sought this room. It was a chamber in many ways strongly characteristic of its owner, a chamber 'like his desires lift upwards and exalt,' but neither wide nor far-penetrating; while its furnishing revealed his fantastic and somewhat childish fancy. At the extremity which faced the door there stood, beneath a crucifix, a small marble altar, on which burned a fire of that strange greenish tinge communicated by certain salts. Except at this extremity, the walls were draped with deep violet curtains bordered by tawny gold, only half displayed by the partial illumination of the place. The light was furnished from lamps of coloured glass, sparsely hung along the length of the room, but numerously clustered about the altar: lamps of diverse tints, amber, peacock-blue, and changefully mingled harmonies of green like the scales on a beetle's back. Above them were coiled thinnest serpentinings of suspended crystal, hued like the tongues in a wintry hearth, flame-colour, voilet, and green; so that, as in the heated current from the lamps the snakes twirled and flickered, and their bright shadows twirled upon the wall, they seemed at length to undulate their twines, and the whole altar became surrounded with a fiery fantasy of sinuous stains.

On the right hand side of the chamber there rose—appearing almost animated in the half lustre—three statues of colossal height, painted to resemble life; for in this matter Florentian followed the taste of the ancient Greeks. They were statues of three poets, and, not insignificantly, of three pagan poets. The first two, Homer and Æschylus, presented no singularity beyond their Titanic proportions; but it was altogether otherwise with the third statue, which was unusual in conception. It was the figure of Virgil; not the Virgil whom *we* know, but the Virgil of mediæval legend, Virgil magician and poet. It bent forwards and downwards towards the spectator; its head was uncircled by any laurel, but on the flowing locks was an impression as of where the wreath had rested; its lowered left hand proffered the magician's rod, its outstretched right poised between light finger-tips the wreath of gilded metal whose impress seemed to linger on its hair: the action was as though it were about to place the laurel on the head of some one beneath. This was the carved embodiment of Florentian's fanatical ambition, a perpetual memento of the double end at which his life was aimed. On the necromancer's rod he could lay his hand, but the laurel of poetic supremacy hung yet beyond his reach. The opposite side of the chamber had but one object to arrest attention: a curious head upon a pedestal, a head of copper with a silver beard, the features not unlike those of a Pan, and the tongue protruded as in derision. This, with a large antique clock, completed the noticeable garniture of the room.

Up and down this apartment Florentian

paced for long, his countenance expressive of inward struggle, till his gaze fell upon the figure of Virgil. His face grew hard; with an air of sudden decision he began to act. Taking from its place the crucifix he threw it on the ground; taking from its pedestal the head he set it on the altar; and it seemed to Florentian as if he reared therewith a demon on the altar of his heart, round which also coiled burning serpents. He sprinkled, in the flame which burned before the head, some drops from a vial; he wounded his arm, and moistened from the wound the idol's tongue, and, stepping back, he set his foot upon the prostrate cross.

A darkness rose like a fountain from the altar, and curled downward through the room as wine through water, until every light was obliterated. Then from out the darkness grew gradually the visage of the idol, soaked with fire; its face was as the planet Mars, its beard as white-hot wire that seethed and crept with heat; and there issued from the lips a voice that threw Florentian on the ground: 'Whom seekest thou?' Twice was the question repeated; and then, as if the display of power were sufficient, the gloom gathered up its edges like a mantle and swept inwards towards the altar; where it settled in a cloud so dense as to eclipse even the visage of fire. A voice came forth again; but a voice that sounded not the same; a voice that seemed to have withered in crossing the confines of existence, and to traverse illimitable remotenesses beyond the imagining of man; a voice melancholy with a boundless calm, the calm not of a crystalline peace but of a marmoreal despair, 'Knowest thou me; what I am?'

Vanity of man! He who had fallen prostrate before this power now rose to his feet with the haughty answer, 'My deity and my slave!'

The unmoved voice held on its way:

'Scarce high enough for thy deity; too high for thy slave, I am pain exceeding great; and the desolation that is at the heart of things, in the barren heath and the barren soul. I am terror without beauty, and force without strength, and sin without delight. I beat my wings against the cope of Eternity, as thou thine against the window of Time. Thou knowest me not, but I know thee, Florentian, what thou art and what thou wouldst. Thou wouldst have and wouldst not give, thou wouldst not render, yet wouldst receive. This cannot be with me. Thou art but half baptized with my baptism, yet wouldst have thy supreme desire. In thine own blood thou wast baptized, and I gave my power to serve thee; thou wouldst have my spirit to inspire thee— thou must be baptized in blood not thine own!'

'Any way but one way!' said Florentian, shuddering.

'One way: no other way. Knowest thou not that in wedding thee to her thou givest me a rival? Thinkest thou my spirit can dwell beside her spirit? Thou must renounce her or me: aye, thou wilt lose not only all thou dreadest to sin for, but all thou hast already sinned for. Render me her body for my temple, and I render thee my spirit to inhabit it. This supreme price thou must pay for thy supreme wish. I ask not her soul. Give that to the God Whom she serves, give her body to me whom thou servest. Why hesitate? It is too late to hesitate, for the time is at hand to act. Choose, before this cloud dissolve which is now dissolving. But remember: thine ambition thou mightest have had; love thou art too deep damned to have.'

The cloud turned from black to grey. ' I consent!' cried Florentian, impetuously.

* * * * *

Three years—what years! since I planted in the grave the laurel which will soon now reach its height; and the fatal memory is heavy upon me, the shadow of my laurel is as the shadow of funeral yew. If confession indeed give ease, I, who am deprived of all other confession, may yet find some appeasement in confessing to this paper. I am not penitent; yet I will do fiercest penance. With the scourge of inexorable recollection I will tear open my scars. With the cuts of a pitiless analysis I make the post-mortem examen of my crime.

Even now can I feel the passions of that moment when (since the forefated hour was not till midnight), leaving her under the influence of the merciful potion which should save *her* from the agony of knowledge and *me* from the agony of knowing that she knew, I sought, in the air of night and in hurrying swiftness, the resolution of which she had deprived me. The glow-worm lamps went out as I sped by, the stars in rainy pools leaped up and went out, too, as if both worm and star were quenched by the shadow of my passing, until I stopped exhausted on the bridge, and looked down into the river. How dark it ran, how deep, how pauseless; how unruffled by a memory of its ancestral hills! Wisely unruffled, perchance. When it first danced down from its native source, did it not predestine all the issues of its current, every darkness through which it should flow, every bough which it should break, every leaf which it should whirl down in its way? Could it, if it would, revoke its waters, and run upward to the holy hills? No; the first step includes all sequent steps; when I did my first evil, I did also this evil; years ago had this shaft been launched, though it was but now curving to its mark; years ago had I smitten her, though she was but now staggering to her fall. Yet I hesitated to act who had already acted, I ruffled my current which I could not draw in. When at length, after long wandering, I retraced my steps, I had not resolved, I had recognized that I could resolve no longer.

She only cried three times. Three times, O my God!—no, not *my* God.

It was close on midnight, and I felt her only, (she was not visible,) as she lay at the feet of Virgil, magician and poet. The lamp had fallen from my hand, and I dared not relume it. I even placed myself between her and the light of the altar, though the salt-green fire was but the spectre of a flame. I reared my arm; I shook; I faltered. At that moment, with a deadly voice, the accomplice-hour gave forth its sinister command.

I swear I struck not the first blow. Some violence seized my hand, and drove the poniard down. Whereat she cried; and I, frenzied, dreading detection, dreading, above all, her wakening,—I struck again, and again she cried; and yet again, and yet again she cried. Then—her eyes opened. I *saw* them open, through the gloom I saw them; through the gloom they were revealed to me, that I might see them to my hour of death. An awful recognition, an unspeakable consciousness grew slowly into them. Motionless with horror they were fixed on mine, motionless with horror mine were fixed on them, as she wakened into death.

How long had I seen them? I saw them still. There was a buzzing in my brain as if a bell had ceased to toll. How long had it ceased to toll? I know not. Has any bell been tolling? I know not. All my senses are resolved into one sense, and that is frozen to those eyes. Silence now, at least; abysmal silence; except the sound (or is the sound in me?), the sound of dripping blood; except that the flame upon the altar sputters, and hisses, and bickers, as if it licked its jaws. Yes, there is another sound—hush, hark!—It is the throbbing of my heart. Not—no, nevermore the throbbing of *her* heart! The loud pulse dies slowly away, as I hope my life is dying; and again I hear the licking of the flame.

A mirror hung opposite to me, and for a second, in some mysterious manner, without ever ceasing to behold the eyes, I beheld also the mirrored flame. The hideous, green, writhing tongue was streaked and flaked with *red!* I swooned, if swoon it can be called; swooned to the mirror, swooned to all about me, swooned to myself, but swooned not to those eyes.

Strange, that no one has taken me, me for such long hours shackled in a gaze! It is night again, is it not? Nay, I remember, I have swooned; what now stirs me from my stupor? Light; the guilty gloom is shuddering at the first sick rays of day. Light? not that, not that; anything but that. Ah! the horrible traitorous light, that will denounce me to myself, that will unshroud to me my dead, that will show me all the monstrous fact. I swooned indeed.

When I recovered consciousness, It was risen from the ground, and kissed me with the kisses of Its mouth.

They told me during the day that the great bell of the cathedral, though no man rang it, had sounded thrice at midnight. It was not a fancy, therefore, that I heard a bell toll *there*, where—when she cried three times. And they asked me jestingly if marriage was ageing me already. I took a mirror to find what they meant. On my forehead were graven three deep wrinkles; and in the locks which fell over my right shoulder I beheld, long and prominent, three white hairs. I carry those marks to this hour. They and a dark stain on the floor at the feet of Virgil are the sole witnesses to that night.

It is three years, I have said, since then; and how have I prospered? Has Tartarus fulfilled its terms of contract, as I faithfully and frightfully fulfilled mine? Yes. In the course which I have driven through every obstacle and every scruple, I have followed at least no phantom-lure. I have risen to the heights of my aspiration, I have overtopped my sole rival. True, it is a tinsel renown; true, Seraphin is still the light-bearer, I but a dragon vomiting infernal fire and smoke which sets the crowd a-gaping. But it is your nature to gape, my good friend of the crowd, and I would have you gape at me. If you prefer to Jove Jove's imitator, what use to be Jove? 'Gods,' you cry; 'what a clatter of swift-footed steeds, and clangour of rapid rolling brazen wheels, and vibrating glare of lamps! Surely, the thunder-maned horses of heaven, the chariot of Olympus; and you must be the mighty Thunderer himself, with the flashing of his awful bolts!' Not so, my short-sighted friend: very laughably otherwise. It is but vain old Salmoneus, gone mad in Elis. I know you, and I know myself. I have what I would have. I work for the present: let Seraphin have the moonshine future, if he lust after it. Present renown means present power; it suffices me that I am supreme in the eyes of my fellow-men. A year since was the laurel decreed to me, and a day ordained for the ceremony: it was only postponed to the present year because of what they thought my calamity. They accounted it calamity, and knew not that it was deliverance. For, my ambition achieved, the compact by which I had achieved it ended, and the demon who had inspired forsook me. Discovery was impossible. A death sudden but natural: how could men know that it was death of the Two-years-dead? I drew breath at length in freedom. For two years It had spoken to me with her lips, used her gestures, smiled her smile:—ingenuity of hell!—for two years the breathing Murder wrought before me, and tortured me in a hundred ways with the living desecration of her form.

Now, relief unspeakable! that vindictive sleuth-hound of my sin has at last lagged from the trail; I have had a year of respite, of release from all torments but those native to my breast; in four days I shall receive the solemn gift of what I already virtually hold; and now, surely, I exult in fruition. If the approach of possession brought not also the approach of recollection, if— Rest, O rest, sad ghost! Is thy grave not deep enough, or the world wide enough, that thou must needs walk the haunted precincts of my heart? Are not spectres there too many, without thee?

Later in the same day. A strange thing has happened to me—if I ought not rather to write a strange nothing. After laying down my pen, I rose and went to the window. I felt the need of some distraction, of escaping from myself. The day, a day in the late autumn, a day of keen winds but bright sunshine, tempted me out: so, putting on cap and mantle, I sallied into the country, where winter pitched his tent on fields yet reddened with the rout of summer. I chose a sheltered lane, whose hedgerows, little visited by the gust, still retained much verdure; and I walked along, gazing with a sense of physical refreshment at the now rare green. As my eyes so wandered, while the mind for a time let slip its care, they were casually caught by the somewhat peculiar trace which a leaf-eating caterpillar had left on one of the leaves. I carelessly outstretched my hand, plucked from the hedge the leaf, and examined it as I strolled. The marking—a large marking which traversed the greater part of the surface—took the shape of a rude but distinct figure, the figure 3. Such a circumstance, thought I, might by a superstitious man be given a personal application; and I fell idly to speculating how it might be applied to myself.

Curious!—I stirred uneasily; I felt my cheek pale, and a chill which was not from the weather creep through me. Three years since *that;* three strokes—three cries—three tolls of the bell—three lines on my brow—three white hairs in my head! I laughed: but the laugh rang false. Then I said, 'Childishness,' threw the leaf away, walked on, hesitated, walked back, picked it up, walked on again, looked at it again. Then, finding I could not laugh myself out of the fancy, I began to reason myself out of it. Even were a supernatural warning probable, a warning refers not to the past but to the future. This referred only to the past, it told me only what I knew already. *Could* it refer to the future? To the bestowal of the laurel? No; that was four days hence, and on the same day was the anniversary of what I feared to name, even in thought. Suddenly I stood still, stabbed to the heart by an idea. I was wrong. The enlaurelling had been postponed to a year from the day on which my supposed affliction was discovered. Now this, although it took place on the day of terrible anniversary, was not known till the day ensuing. Consequently, though it wanted four days to the bestowal of the laurel, it lacked but three days to the date of my crime. The chain of coincidence was complete. I dropped the leaf as if it had death in it, and strove to evade, by rapid motion and thinking of other things, the idea which appalled me. But, as a man walking in a mist circles continually to the point from which he started, so, in whatever direction I turned the footsteps of my mind, they wandered back to that unabandonable thought. I returned trembling to the house.

Of course it is nothing; a mere coincidence, that is all. Yes; a mere coincidence, perhaps, if it had been *one* coincidence. But when it is seven coincidences! Three stabs, three cries, three tolls, three lines, three hairs, three years, three days; and on the very date when these coincidences meet, the key to them is put into my hands by the casual work of an insect on a casual leaf, casually plucked. This day alone of all days in my life the scattered rays converge; they are instantly focussed and flashed on my mind by a leaf! It may be a coincidence, only a coincidence; but it is a coincidence at which my marrow sets. I will write no further till the day comes. If by that time anything has happened to confirm my dread, I will record what has chanced.

One thing broods over me with the oppression of certainty. If this incident be indeed a warning that but three days stand as barriers between me and nearing justice, then doom will come upon me at the unforgettable minute when it came on her.

The third day.—It is an hour before midnight, and I sit in my room of statues. I dare not sleep if I could sleep; and I write, because the rushing thoughts move slower through the turnstile of expression. I have chosen this place to make what may be my last vigil and last notes, partly from obedience to an inexplicable yet comprehensible fascination, partly from a deliberate resolve. I would face the lightning of vengeance on the very spot where I most tempt its stroke, that if it strike not I may cease to fear its striking. Here then I sit to tease with final questioning the Sibyl of my destiny. With *final* questioning; for never since the fisrt shock have I ceased to question her, nor she to return me riddling answers. She unrolls her volume till my sight and heart ache at it together. I have been struck by innumerable deaths; I have perished under a fresh doom every day, every hour—in these last hours, every minute. I write in black thought; and tear, as soon as written, guess after guess at fate till the floor of my brain is littered with them.

That the deed has been discovered—that seems to me most probable, that is the conjecture which oftenest recurs. Appallingly probable! Yet how improbable, could I only reason it. Aye, but I cannot reason it. What reason will be left me, if I survive this hour?

What, indeed, have I to do with reason, or has reason to do with this, where all is beyond reason, where the very foundation of my dread is unassailable simply because it is unreasonable? What crime can be interred so cunningly, but it will toss in its grave, and tumble the sleeked earth above it? Or some hidden witness may have beheld me, or the prudently-kept imprudence of this writing may have encountered some unsuspected eye. In any case the issue is the same; the hour which struck down her will also strike down me: I shall perish on the scaffold or at the stake, unaided by my occult powers; for I serve a master who is the prince of cowards, and can fight only from ambush. Be it by these ways, or by any of the countless intricacies that my restless mind has unravelled, the vengeance will come: its occasion may be an accident of the instant, a wandering mote of chance; but the vengeance is pre-ordained and inevitable. When the Alpine avalanche is poised for descent, the most trivial cause—a casual shout—will suffice to start the loosened ruin on its way; and so the mere echoes of the clock that beats out midnight will disintegrate upon me the precipitant wrath.

Repent? Nay, nay, it could not have been otherwise than it was; the defile was close behind me, I could but go forward, forward. If I was merciless to her, was I not more merciless to myself; could I hesitate to sacrifice her life, who did not hesitate to sacrifice my soul? I do not repent, I cannot repent; it is a thing for inconsequent weaklings. To repent your purposes is comprehensible, to repent your deeds most futile. To shake the tree, and then not gather the fruit—a fool's act! Aye, but if the fruit be not worth the gathering? If this fame was not worth the sinning for—this fame, with the multitude's clapping hands half-drowned by the growl of winds that comes in gusts through the unbarred gate of hell? If I am miserable with it, and might have been happy without it? With her, without ambition—yes, it might have been. Wife and child! I have more in my heart than I have hitherto written. I have an intermittent pang of loss. Yes, I, murderer, worse than murderer, have still passions that are not deadly, but tender.

I met a child to-day; a child with great candour of eyes. They who talk of children's instincts are at fault: she knew not that hell was in my soul, she knew only that softness was in my gaze. She had been gathering wild flowers, and offered them to me. To me, to *me!* I was inexpressibly touched and pleased, curiously touched and pleased. I spoke to her gently, and with open confidence she began to talk. Heaven knows it was little enough she talked of! Commonest common things, pettiest childish things, fondest foolish things. Of her school, her toys, the strawberries in her garden, her little brothers and sisters—nothing, surely,

to interest any man. Yet I listened enchanted.
How simple it all was; how strange, how wonderful, how sweet! And she knew not that my
eyes were anhungered of her, she knew not that
my ears were gluttonous of her speech, she could
not have understood it had I told her; none
could, none. For all this exquisiteness is among
the commonplaces of life to other men, like the
raiment they indue at rising, like the bread
they weary of eating, like the daisies they trample under blind feet; knowing not what raiment is to him who has felt the ravening wind,
knowing not what bread is to him who has
lacked all bread, knowing not what daisies are
to him whose feet have wandered in grime.
How can these elves be to such men what
they are to me, who am damned to the eternal
loss of them? Why was I never told that the
laurel could soothe no hunger, that the laurel
could staunch no pang, that the laurel could
return no kiss? But needed I to be told it, did
I not know it? Yes, my brain knew it, my
heart knew it not. And now——.

At half-past eleven.

O lente, lente currite, noctis equi!

Just! they are the words of that other trafficker
in his own soul.* Me, like him, the time
tracks swiftly down; I can fly no farther, I fall

* Faustus, in the last scene of Marlowe's play.

exhausted, the fanged hour fastens on my throat: they will break into the room, my guilt will burst its grave and point at me; I shall be seized, I shall be condemned, I shall be executed; I shall be no longer I, but a nameless lump on which they pasture worms. Or perhaps the hour will herald some yet worser thing, some sudden death, some undreamable, ghastly surprise—ah! what is that at the door there, that, that with *her* eyes? Nothing: the door is shut. Surely, surely, I am not to die now? Destiny steals upon a man asleep or off his guard, not when he is awake, as I am awake, at watch, as I am at watch, wide-eyed, vigilant, alert. Oh, miserable hope! Watch the eaves of your house, to bar the melting of the snow; or guard the gateways of the clouds, to bar the forthgoing of the lightning; or guard the four quarters of the heavens, to bar the way of the winds: but what prescient hand can close the Hecatompyloi of fate, what might arrest the hurrying retributions whose multitudinous tramplings converge upon me in a hundred presages, in a hundred shrivelling menaces, down all the echoing avenues of doom? It is but a question of which shall arrive the fleetest and the first. I cease to think. I am all a waiting and a fear. *Twelve!*

At half-past two. Midnight is stricken, and I am unstricken. Guilt, indeed, makes babies of the wisest. Nothing happened; absolutely nothing. For two hours I watched with lessening expectance: still nothing. I laughed aloud between sudden light-heartedness and scorn. Ineffable fool that I was, I had conjured up death, judgement, doom—heaven knows what, all because a caterpillar had crawled along a leaf! And then, as I might have done before had not terror vitiated my reason, I made essay whether I still retained my power. I retain it. Let me set down for my own enhardiment what the oracle replied to my questioning.

'Have I not promised and kept my promise, shall I not promise and keep? You would be crowned and you shall be crowned. Does your way to achievement lie through misery?—is not that the way to all worth the achieving? Are not half the mill-wheels of the world turned by waters of pain? Mountain summit that would rise into the clouds, can you not suffer the eternal snows? If your heart fail you, turn; I chain you not. I will restore you your oath. I will cancel your bond. Go to the God Who has tenderness for such weaklings: *my* service requires the strong.'

What a slave of my fancy was I! Excellent fool, what! pay the forfeit of my sin and forgo the recompense, recoil from the very gates of conquest? I fear no longer: the crisis is past, the day of promise has begun, I go forward to my destiny; I triumph.

* * * * *

Florentian laid down his pen, and passed into dreams. He saw the crowd, the throne, the waiting laurel, the sunshine, the flashing of rich robes; he heard the universal shout of acclaim, he felt the flush of intoxicating pride. He rose, his form dilating with exultation, and passed, lamp in hand, to the foot of the third statue. The colossal figure leaned above him with its outstretched laurel, its proffered wand, its melancholy face and flowing hair; so lifelike was it that in the wavering flame of the lamp the laurel seemed to move. 'At length, Virgil,' said Florentian, 'at length I am equal with you; Virgil, magician and poet, your crown shall descend on me!'

One.. Two.. Three! The strokes of the great clock shook the chamber, shook the statues; and after the strokes had ceased, the echoes were still prolonged. Was it only an echo?

Boom!

Or—*was it the cathedral bell?*

Boom!

It *was* the cathedral bell. Yet a third time, sombre, surly, ominous as the bay of a nearing bloodhound, the sound came down the wind.

Boom!

Horror clutched his heart. He looked up at the statue. He turned to fly. But a few hairs, tangled round the lowered wand, for a single instant held him like a cord. He knew, without seeing, that they were the three white hairs.

When, later in the day, a deputation of officials came to escort Florentian to the place fixed for his coronation, they were informed that he had been all night in his Chamber of Statues, nor had he yet made his appearance. They waited while the servant left to fetch him. The man was away some time, and they talked gaily as they waited: a bird beat its wings at the window; through the open door came in a stream of sunlight, and the fragmentary song of a young girl passing:

> Oh, syne she tripped, and syne she ran
> (The water-lily's a lightsome flower),
> All for joy and sunshine weather
> The lily and Marjorie danced together,
> As he came down from Langley Tower.
>
> There's a blackbird sits on Langley Tower,
> And a throstle on Glenlindy's tree;
> The throstle sings ' Robin, my heart's love! '
> And the blackbird, ' Bonnie, sweet Marjorie! '

The man came running back at last, with a blanched face and a hushed voice. ' Come,' he said, ' and see! '

They went and saw.

At the feet of Virgil's statue Florentian lay dead. A dark pool almost hid that dark stain on the ground, the three lines on his forehead were etched in blood, and across the shattered brow lay a ponderous gilded wreath; while over the extinguished altar-fire the idol seemed to quiver its derisive tongue.

'He is already laurelled,' said one, breaking at length the silence; 'we come too late.'

Too late. The crown of Virgil, magician and poet, had descended on him.

MICHIGAN
CHRISTIAN
COLLEGE
LIBRARY
ROCHESTER, MICH.

ENNIS AND NANCY HAM LIBRARY
ROCHESTER COLLEGE
800 WEST AVON ROAD
ROCHE